T0280743

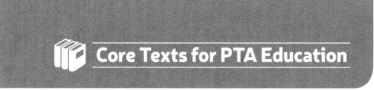

Core Texts for PTA Education

Entry-Level Skill Checklists
for Physical Therapist Assistant Students

SERIES EDITOR

MIA L. ERICKSON, PT, EDD, CHT, ATC

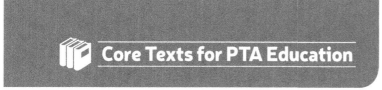
Core Texts for PTA Education

Entry-Level Skill Checklists
for Physical Therapist Assistant Students

Terry Larson, PT, DPT

Program Director
Physical Therapist Assistant Program
Community Based Education & Development (CBD College)
Los Angeles, California

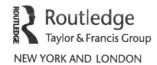
Routledge
Taylor & Francis Group

NEW YORK AND LONDON

First published in 2023 by SLACK Incorporated

Published in 2024 by Routledge
605 Third Avenue, New York, NY 10158

and by Routledge
4 Park Square, Milton Park, Abingdon, Oxon, OX14 4RN

Routledge is an imprint of the Taylor & Francis Group, an informa business

© 2023 Taylor & Francis Group

Dr. Terry Larson *reported no financial or proprietary interest in the materials presented herein.*

Cover Artist: Tinhouse Design

Library of Congress Control Number: 2022951960

ISBN: 9781630919986 (pbk)
ISBN: 9781003523987 (ebk)

DOI: 10.4324/9781003523987

CONTENTS

ABOUT THE AUTHOR

Terry Larson, PT, DPT, completed a Bachelor of Arts in Dance (2000), a Master of Science in Physical Therapy (2004), and a Doctorate in Physical Therapy from the University of St. Augustine (2008). She owns a private in-home pelvic health practice in Florida, treating men and women with pelvic floor dysfunction and associated orthopedic conditions. She is the Program Director for the Hybrid Physical Therapist Assistant Program at Community Based Education & Development (CBD College) in Los Angeles, California. In addition, she is a Senior Teaching Assistant for Herman and Wallace Pelvic Health Institute and Associated Faculty for Hanover College, Bowling Green State University, South College, and Augustana College Hybrid DPT programs.

PREFACE

As a physical therapist assistant program faculty member, I began to get frustrated with creating and recreating skill checklists. As a program director, I struggled with ensuring all faculty were on the same page with skill checks and that all students knew exactly what to expect during the assessment. I decided to streamline the process and create a study guide for the students and an easy tool for instructors to utilize during grading. I developed these checklists to simplify the process and guarantee that any instructor who assesses a skill is looking for the same level of performance. The skill checklists in this book are the culmination of years of updating and perfecting the checklist document.

This book was written to accompany a physical therapist assistant student throughout their academic program. My intention is for the student to use this lab manual throughout the program in all courses. Using this book, the process of skill checks hopefully will be less cumbersome for the faculty and student. Each student should be provided a lab book on day one of the program and use it to house their completed skill checks throughout the program. At the end of the program, the student can submit the manual as documentation that they have passed all required entry-level skills of a physical therapist assistant. Based on your school policies, you could collect them at the end to store for compliance.

Section I

Data Collection

Chapter 1

Vital Signs

Larson T. *Entry-Level Skill Checklists for
Physical Therapist Assistant Students* (pp 3-6).
© 2023 Taylor & Francis Group.

Student Name: _____

Skill		Vital Signs			
Source		Memolo J. *Procedures and Patient Care for the Physical Therapist Assistant.* SLACK Incorporated; 2019.	**Check When Completed**		
			Self	Peer	Instructor
Student Introduction and Consent	1 ⚑	The student introduces themself to the patient. Must include that they are a **student** PTA and list the school's name.	☐	☐	☐
	2 ⚑	The student verifies the patient's identity. Must use at least 2 patient identifiers (name, date of birth).	☐	☐	☐
	3 ⚑	The student gains consent: • Speaks with the patient about their status (acquires relevant information) • Educates the patient on intended data collection/intervention and goals for the session • Gains permission to perform said data collection/intervention	☐	☐	☐
Student, Patient, and Supply Preparation	4 ⚑	The student gathers supplies and prepares treatment area (cleans equipment, checks for safety hazards, ensures all equipment is functional and appropriate).	☐	☐	☐
	5	The student washes their hands:			
		Student removes all jewelry from their wrists and hands. Student turns the water to the preferred temperature and wets their hands. Student applies the soap to their hands and washes them with their hands pointed down. Student scrubs for 40–60 seconds and includes palm, between fingers, fingernails, and dorsum of hands. Student rinses hands with hands pointed down. Student dries their hands with a paper towel, uses a paper towel to turn off the water, and then disposes of the paper towel in the trash.	☐	☐	☐
	6	The student places the patient in the correct position for support, comfort, and access to body area necessary for data collection/intervention.	☐	☐	☐
Skill Performance	7	The student correctly measures the patient's **Heart Rate (radial artery)**:			
		Student correctly locates patient's radial artery by palpating the radial styloid at the base of the thumb with their first 2 fingers. Student then moves their fingers slightly medial.	☐	☐	☐
		Student counts the beats silently for 1 full minute.	☐	☐	☐
		Student records the heart rate in beats/minute and notes rhythm and volume.	☐	☐	☐
	8	The student correctly measures the patient's **Heart Rate (carotid artery)**:			
		Student correctly locates patient's carotid artery by sliding their first 2 fingers down the length of patient's jaw about 2 inches, just starting at the base of the ear. Student then slides the fingers just inferior to the jawbone and anterior to the sternocleidomastoid muscle.	☐	☐	☐
		Student counts the beats silently for 1 full minute.	☐	☐	☐
		Student records the heart rate in beats/minute and notes rhythm and volume.	☐	☐	☐
		Student correctly states the normal resting heart rate ranges for adults, children, infants, and athletes: *(Adult: 60–100 beats/minute Children: 85–205 beats/minute Infants: 100–190 beats/minute Athletes: 40–60 beats/minute).*	☐	☐	☐

⚑ = Critical Safety Element/Professionalism. If a student is unable to complete a flagged step without cueing, they will need to return at another time to redo the check-off. All other steps can be cued.

	9	The student correctly measures the patient's **Respiratory Rate**:			
		Student simulates the measurement of the radial pulse while resting patient's arm on their thorax.	☐	☐	☐
		Student counts either inspirations or expirations for 1 minute.	☐	☐	☐
		Student records the respiratory rate in breaths/minute and notes rhythm, depth, and character of respirations.	☐	☐	☐
		Student correctly states the normal respiratory heart rate ranges for adults, infants, and children: *(Adult: 12–16 breaths/minute Children: 18–30 breaths/minute Infants: 30–60 breaths/minute).*	☐	☐	☐
	10	The student correctly measures the patient's **Oxygen Saturation**:			
		Student places the oximeter over patient's fingertip. If patient has nail polish, remove it. If their hands are cold, warm them up before application.	☐	☐	☐
		Student keeps the oximeter on patient's finger for 1 minute before recording the reading.	☐	☐	☐
		Student records the oxygen saturation in percentage (SpO_2).	☐	☐	☐
		Student correctly states the normal oxygen saturation rate: *(SpO_2: 95%–100%).*	☐	☐	☐
	11	The student correctly measures the patient's **Blood Pressure**:			
		Student seats patient with the left upper extremity supported on a table (or another surface) at heart level.	☐	☐	☐
		Student asks patient to remove any clothing in the area before applying the cuff.	☐	☐	☐
		Student places the cuff approximately 1 inch superior to the antecubital space ensuring the gauge can easily be seen and read.	☐	☐	☐
		Student determines the inflation number by palpating the radial pulse while inflating the cuff to 70–80 mm Hg, continuing to inflate until the radial pulse is no longer palpable. Continue to inflate to 30 mm Hg above the number at which you can no longer palpate the radial pulse.	☐	☐	☐
		Student deflates the cuff and has patient rest for 30–60 seconds.	☐	☐	☐
		Student places the stethoscope bell over the brachial artery and listens for a pulse. Once the pulse is confirmed, reinflate the cuff to the number 30 mm Hg over the number at which the radial pulse was not palpable.	☐	☐	☐
		Student listens for the Korotkoff sounds and notes the readings.	☐	☐	☐
		Student records the blood pressure as mm Hg as well as patient's position and extremity used.	☐	☐	☐
		Student correctly states the normal resting blood pressure for adults, HTN stage 1, 2, and hypertensive crisis: *(Adults: <120/80 mm Hg HTN stage 1: 130–139/80–89 mm Hg HTN stage 2: >140/90 mm Hg Hypertensive crisis: >180/120 mm Hg).*	☐	☐	☐
Post-Skill	12	The student washes their hands post–skill performance:			
		Student removes all jewelry from their wrists and hands. Student turns the water to the preferred temperature and wets their hands. Student applies the soap to their hands and washes them with their hands pointed down. Student scrubs for 40–60 seconds and includes palm, between fingers, fingernails, and dorsum of hands. Student rinses hands with hands pointed down. Student dries their hands with a paper towel, uses a paper towel to turn off the water, and then disposes of the paper towel in the trash.	☐	☐	☐
	13	The student verbalizes that they will document their session in the note.	☐	☐	☐

⚐ = Critical Safety Element/Professionalism. If a student is unable to complete a flagged step without cueing, they will need to return at another time to redo the check-off. All other steps can be cued.

Other	14 ⚑	The student has optimal body mechanics during performance of the skill.		☐	☐	☐
	15 ⚑	The student uses appropriate therapeutic touch.		☐	☐	☐
	16	The student is able to complete the check-off in the time allotted.		☐	☐	☐
Communication	17	The student uses language the patient can understand.		☐	☐	☐
	18	The student listens actively to the patient during the session.		☐	☐	☐
	19	The student ensures the patient understands instructions by having the patient teach back or demonstrate.		☐	☐	☐
	20 ⚑	The student demonstrates confidence and provides the patient with clear instruction and cueing.		☐	☐	☐
Peer Name (Printed)			**Peer Signature**		**Date of Peer Review**	
Instructor Name (Printed and Signature)	By signing this skills checklist, I am declaring this student competent in the skill described above.				**Date of Instructor Review**	
NOTES						

⚑ = Critical Safety Element/Professionalism. If a student is unable to complete a flagged step without cueing, they will need to return at another time to redo the check-off. All other steps can be cued.

Chapter 2
Gait and Balance Testing

Larson T. *Entry-Level Skill Checklists for*
Physical Therapist Assistant Students (pp 7-17).
© 2023 Taylor & Francis Group.

Student Name: _____

Skill		Gait and Balance Testing: Tinetti Test/Performance-Oriented Mobility Assessment			
Source		Memolo J. *Procedures and Patient Care for the Physical Therapist Assistant.* SLACK Incorporated; 2019.	**Check When Completed**		
			Self	Peer	Instructor
Student Introduction and Consent	1 ⚑	The student introduces themself to the patient. Must include that they are a **student** PTA and list the school's name.	☐	☐	☐
	2 ⚑	The student verifies the patient's identity. Must use at least 2 patient identifiers (name, date of birth).	☐	☐	☐
	3 ⚑	The student gains consent: • Speaks with the patient about their status (acquires relevant information) • Educates the patient on intended data collection/intervention and goals for the session • Gains permission to perform said data collection/intervention	☐	☐	☐
Student, Patient, and Supply Preparation	4 ⚑	The student gathers supplies and prepares treatment area (cleans equipment, checks for safety hazards, ensures all equipment is functional and appropriate).	☐	☐	☐
	5	The student washes their hands:			
		Student removes all jewelry from their wrists and hands. Student turns the water to the preferred temperature and wets their hands. Student applies the soap to their hands and washes them with their hands pointed down. Student scrubs for 40–60 seconds and includes palm, between fingers, fingernails, and dorsum of hands. Student rinses hands with hands pointed down. Student dries their hands with a paper towel, uses a paper towel to turn off the water, and then disposes of the paper towel in the trash.	☐	☐	☐
	6	The student places the patient in the correct position for support, comfort, and access to body area necessary for data collection/intervention.	☐	☐	☐
	7	The student applies gait belt safely and securely to the patient.	☐	☐	☐
Skill Performance	8	The student correctly performs the **Tinetti Test**:			
		Student correctly explains testing process to patient: *(This test is going to assess gait and balance during different activities).*	☐	☐	☐
		Student correctly performs the test.	☐	☐	☐
		Student provides appropriate guarding techniques. Preferred assistive device is permitted.	☐	☐	☐
		Student determines test score and explains the results: *(18 or less = high risk for falls 19–23 = moderate risk for falls 24 or higher = low risk for falls).*	☐	☐	☐

⚑ = Critical Safety Element/Professionalism. If a student is unable to complete a flagged step without cueing, they will need to return at another time to redo the check-off. All other steps can be cued.

	9	The student washes their hands post–skill performance:			
Post-Skill		Student removes all jewelry from their wrists and hands. Student turns the water to the preferred temperature and wets their hands. Student applies the soap to their hands and washes them with their hands pointed down. Student scrubs for 40–60 seconds and includes palm, between fingers, fingernails, and dorsum of hands. Student rinses hands with hands pointed down. Student dries their hands with a paper towel, uses a paper towel to turn off the water, and then disposes of the paper towel in the trash.	☐	☐	☐
	10	The student verbalizes that they will document their session in the note.	☐	☐	☐
Other	11 ⚑	The student has optimal body mechanics during performance of the skill.	☐	☐	☐
	12 ⚑	The student uses appropriate therapeutic touch.	☐	☐	☐
	13	The student is able to complete the check-off in the time allotted.	☐	☐	☐
Communication	14	The student uses language the patient can understand.	☐	☐	☐
	15	The student listens actively to the patient during the session.	☐	☐	☐
	16	The student ensures the patient understands instructions by having the patient teach back or demonstrate.	☐	☐	☐
	17 ⚑	The student demonstrates confidence and provides the patient with clear instruction and cueing.	☐	☐	☐

Peer Name (Printed)		Peer Signature		Date of Peer Review	
Instructor Name (Printed and Signature)	By signing this skills checklist, I am declaring this student competent in the skill described above.			Date of Instructor Review	
NOTES					

⚑ = Critical Safety Element/Professionalism. If a student is unable to complete a flagged step without cueing, they will need to return at another time to redo the check-off. All other steps can be cued.

Tinetti Performance-Oriented Mobility Assessment

Description: The Tinetti assessment tool is an easily administered, task-oriented test that measures an older adult's gait and balance abilities.
Equipment needed: Hard, armless chair; stopwatch or wristwatch; 15-foot walkway.
Completion time: 10–15 minutes.
Scoring: A 3-point ordinal scale ranging from 0–2. Zero indicates the highest level of impairment and 2 indicates the individual's independence.

Balance Tests

Initial instructions: Patient is seated in hard, armless chair. The following maneuvers are tested:

Sitting Balance	Leans or slides in chair	0	
	Steady, safe	1	
Arises	Unable without help	0	
	Able, uses arms to help	1	
	Able without using arms	2	
Attempts to Arise	Unable without help	0	
	Able, requires more than 1 attempt	1	
	Able, 1 attempt	2	
Immediate Standing Balance (First 5 seconds)	Unsteady (swaggers, moves feet, trunk sway)	0	
	Steady but uses walker or other support	1	
	Steady without walker or other support	2	
Standing Balance	Unsteady	0	
	Steady but wide stance (medial heels more than 4 inches apart) AND uses cane or other support	1	
	Narrow stance without support	2	
Nudged (Patient at maximum position with feet as close together as possible, examiner pushes lightly on patient's sternum with palm of hand 3 times)	Begins to fall	0	
	Staggers, grabs, catches self	1	
	Steady	2	
Eyes Closed (At maximum position)	Unsteady	0	
	Steady	1	
Turning 360 Degrees—Steps	Discontinuous steps	0	
	Continuous steps	1	
Turning 360 Degrees—Steadiness	Unsteady (staggers, grabs)	0	
	Steady	1	
Sitting Down	Unsafe (misjudged distance, falls into chair)	0	
	Uses arms or unsmooth motion	1	
	Safe, smooth motion	2	
	Total (Balance Score):	/16	

⬜ = Critical Safety Element/Professionalism. If a student is unable to complete a flagged step without cueing, they will need to return at another time to redo the check-off. All other steps can be cued.

Gait Tests

Initial instructions: Patient stands with examiner, walks down hallway or across room, first at "usual" pace, then back to "rapid, but safe" pace (using usual walking aids).

Initiation of Gait (Immediately after told to "go")	Any hesitancy or multiple attempts to start	0	
	No hesitancy	1	
Step Length (Right swing foot)	Does not pass left stance foot with step	0	
	Passes left stance foot	1	
Step Height (Right swing foot)	Right foot does not clear floor completely with step	0	
	Right foot completely clears floor	1	
Step Length (Left swing foot)	Does not pass right stance foot with step	0	
	Passes right stance foot	1	
Step Height (Left swing foot)	Left foot does not clear floor completely with step	0	
	Left foot completely clears floor	1	
Step Symmetry	Right and left step length not equal (estimated)	0	
	Right and left step length appear equal	1	
Step Continuity	Stopping or discontinuity between steps	0	
	Steps appear continuous	1	
Path (Estimated in relation to floor tiles, 12-inch diameter; observe excursion of 1 foot over about 10 feet of the course)	Marked deviation	0	
	Mild/moderate deviation OR uses walking aid	1	
	Straight without walking aid	2	
Trunk	Marked sway OR uses walking aid	0	
	No sway but flexion of knees or back or spreads arms out while walking	1	
	No sway, no flexion, no use of arms, and no use of walking aid	2	
Walking Stance	Heels apart	0	
	Heels almost touching while walking	1	
	Total (Gait Score):		/12
Total POMA Score (Gait Score + Balance Score)	/28		

⌐ = Critical Safety Element/Professionalism. If a student is unable to complete a flagged step without cueing, they will need to return at another time to redo the check-off. All other steps can be cued.

Student Name: _____

Skill		Gait and Balance Testing: Timed Up and Go Test			
Source		Memolo J. *Procedures and Patient Care for the Physical Therapist Assistant.* SLACK Incorporated; 2019.	**Check When Completed**		
			Self	Peer	Instructor
Student Introduction and Consent	1 ⚑	The student introduces themself to the patient. Must include that they are a **student** PTA and list the school's name.	☐	☐	☐
	2 ⚑	The student verifies the patient's identity. Must use at least 2 patient identifiers (name, date of birth).	☐	☐	☐
	3 ⚑	The student gains consent: • Speaks with the patient about their status (acquires relevant information) • Educates the patient on intended data collection/intervention and goals for the session • Gains permission to perform said data collection/intervention	☐	☐	☐
Student, Patient, and Supply Preparation	4 ⚑	The student gathers supplies and prepares treatment area (cleans equipment, checks for safety hazards, ensures all equipment is functional and appropriate).	☐	☐	☐
	5	The student washes their hands:			
		Student removes all jewelry from their wrists and hands. Student turns the water to the preferred temperature and wets their hands. Student applies the soap to their hands and washes them with their hands pointed down. Student scrubs for 40–60 seconds and includes palm, between fingers, fingernails, and dorsum of hands. Student rinses hands with hands pointed down. Student dries their hands with a paper towel, uses a paper towel to turn off the water, and then disposes of the paper towel in the trash.	☐	☐	☐
	6	The student places the patient in the correct position for support, comfort, and access to body area necessary for data collection/intervention.	☐	☐	☐
	7	The student applies gait belt safely and securely to the patient.	☐	☐	☐
Skill Performance	8	The student correctly performs the **Timed Up and Go Test**:			
		Student correctly sets up testing area: *(Measures out 3 meters from the chair where patient will sit).*	☐	☐	☐
		Student correctly explains testing purpose to patient: *(This test is going to assess your mobility).*	☐	☐	☐
		Student correctly performs the test: *(When I say "go," I would like you to stand up, walk to the marked location, turn around, return to the chair, and sit again).*	☐	☐	☐
		Student provides appropriate guarding techniques. Preferred assistive device is permitted.	☐	☐	☐
		Student starts a timer when they say "go" and stops the time when patient returns to the chair.	☐	☐	☐
		Student determines test score and explains the results: *(>30 seconds = very high risk for falls* *12–30 seconds = high risk for falls).*	☐	☐	☐
Post-Skill	9	The student washes their hands post–skill performance:			
		Student removes all jewelry from their wrists and hands. Student turns the water to the preferred temperature and wets their hands. Student applies the soap to their hands and washes them with their hands pointed down. Student scrubs for 40–60 seconds and includes palm, between fingers, fingernails, and dorsum of hands. Student rinses hands with hands pointed down. Student dries their hands with a paper towel, uses a paper towel to turn off the water, and then disposes of the paper towel in the trash.	☐	☐	☐
	10	The student verbalizes that they will document their session in the note.	☐	☐	☐

⚑ = Critical Safety Element/Professionalism. If a student is unable to complete a flagged step without cueing, they will need to return at another time to redo the check-off. All other steps can be cued.

Other	11 ⚑	The student has optimal body mechanics during performance of the skill.	☐	☐	☐
	12 ⚑	The student uses appropriate therapeutic touch.	☐	☐	☐
	13	The student is able to complete the check-off in the time allotted.	☐	☐	☐
Communication	14	The student uses language the patient can understand.	☐	☐	☐
	15	The student listens actively to the patient during the session.	☐	☐	☐
	16	The student ensures the patient understands instructions by having the patient teach back or demonstrate.	☐	☐	☐
	17 ⚑	The student demonstrates confidence and provides the patient with clear instruction and cueing.	☐	☐	☐
Peer Name (Printed)			**Peer Signature**		**Date of Peer Review**	
Instructor Name (Printed and Signature)	By signing this skills checklist, I am declaring this student competent in the skill described above.			**Date of Instructor Review**	
NOTES					

⚑ = Critical Safety Element/Professionalism. If a student is unable to complete a flagged step without cueing, they will need to return at another time to redo the check-off. All other steps can be cued.

Student Name: _____

Skill		Gait and Balance Testing: Berg Balance Scale			
Source		Memolo J. *Procedures and Patient Care for the Physical Therapist Assistant.* SLACK Incorporated; 2019.	**Check When Completed**		
			Self	Peer	Instructor
Student Introduction and Consent	1 ⚑	The student introduces themself to the patient. Must include that they are a **student** PTA and list the school's name.	☐	☐	☐
	2 ⚑	The student verifies the patient's identity. Must use at least 2 patient identifiers (name, date of birth).	☐	☐	☐
	3 ⚑	The student gains consent: • Speaks with the patient about their status (acquires relevant information) • Educates the patient on intended data collection/intervention and goals for the session • Gains permission to perform said data collection/intervention	☐	☐	☐
Student, Patient, and Supply Preparation	4 ⚑	The student gathers supplies and prepares treatment area (cleans equipment, checks for safety hazards, ensures all equipment is functional and appropriate).	☐	☐	☐
	5	The student washes their hands:			
		Student removes all jewelry from their wrists and hands. Student turns the water to the preferred temperature and wets their hands. Student applies the soap to their hands and washes them with their hands pointed down. Student scrubs for 40–60 seconds and includes palm, between fingers, fingernails, and dorsum of hands. Student rinses hands with hands pointed down. Student dries their hands with a paper towel, uses a paper towel to turn off the water, and then disposes of the paper towel in the trash.	☐	☐	☐
	6	The student places the patient in the correct position for support, comfort, and access to body area necessary for data collection/intervention.	☐	☐	☐
	7	The student applies gait belt safely and securely to the patient.	☐	☐	☐
Skill Performance	8	The student correctly performs the **Berg Balance Scale**:			
		Student correctly explains testing purpose to patient: *(This test is going to assess your ability to perform everyday tasks).*	☐	☐	☐
		Student correctly performs the test.	☐	☐	☐
		Student provides appropriate guarding techniques. Assistive device is NOT permitted.	☐	☐	☐
		Student determines test score and explains the results: *(0–20 = high risk for falls* *21–40 = moderate risk for falls* *41–56 = low risk for falls).*	☐	☐	☐
Post-Skill	9	The student washes their hands post–skill performance:			
		Student removes all jewelry from their wrists and hands. Student turns the water to the preferred temperature and wets their hands. Student applies the soap to their hands and washes them with their hands pointed down. Student scrubs for 40–60 seconds and includes palm, between fingers, fingernails, and dorsum of hands. Student rinses hands with hands pointed down. Student dries their hands with a paper towel, uses a paper towel to turn off the water, and then disposes of the paper towel in the trash.	☐	☐	☐
	10	The student verbalizes that they will document their session in the note.	☐	☐	☐
Other	11 ⚑	The student has optimal body mechanics during performance of the skill.	☐	☐	☐
	12 ⚑	The student uses appropriate therapeutic touch.	☐	☐	☐
	13	The student is able to complete the check-off in the time allotted.	☐	☐	☐

⚑ = Critical Safety Element/Professionalism. If a student is unable to complete a flagged step without cueing, they will need to return at another time to redo the check-off. All other steps can be cued.

Communication	14	The student uses language the patient can understand.	☐	☐	☐
	15	The student listens actively to the patient during the session.	☐	☐	☐
	16	The student ensures the patient understands instructions by having the patient teach back or demonstrate.	☐	☐	☐
	17 ⚑	The student demonstrates confidence and provides the patient with clear instruction and cueing.	☐	☐	☐

Peer Name (Printed)		Peer Signature		Date of Peer Review	
Instructor Name (Printed and Signature)	By signing this skills checklist, I am declaring this student competent in the skill described above.			Date of Instructor Review	
NOTES					

⚑ = Critical Safety Element/Professionalism. If a student is unable to complete a flagged step without cueing, they will need to return at another time to redo the check-off. All other steps can be cued.

Student Name: _____

Skill		Gait and Balance Testing: Dynamic Gait Index			
Source		Memolo J. *Procedures and Patient Care for the Physical Therapist Assistant.* SLACK Incorporated; 2019.	**Check When Completed**		
			Self	Peer	Instructor
Student Introduction and Consent	1 ⚑	The student introduces themself to the patient. Must include that they are a **student** PTA and list the school's name.	☐	☐	☐
	2 ⚑	The student verifies the patient's identity. Must use at least 2 patient identifiers (name, date of birth).	☐	☐	☐
	3 ⚑	The student gains consent: • Speaks with the patient about their status (acquires relevant information) • Educates the patient on intended data collection/intervention and goals for the session • Gains permission to perform said data collection/intervention	☐	☐	☐
Student, Patient, and Supply Preparation	4 ⚑	The student gathers supplies and prepares treatment area (cleans equipment, checks for safety hazards, ensures all equipment is functional and appropriate).	☐	☐	☐
	5	The student washes their hands:			
		Student removes all jewelry from their wrists and hands. Student turns the water to the preferred temperature and wets their hands. Student applies the soap to their hands and washes them with their hands pointed down. Student scrubs for 40–60 seconds and includes palm, between fingers, fingernails, and dorsum of hands. Student rinses hands with hands pointed down. Student dries their hands with a paper towel, uses a paper towel to turn off the water, and then disposes of the paper towel in the trash.	☐	☐	☐
	6	The student places the patient in the correct position for support, comfort, and access to body area necessary for data collection/intervention.	☐	☐	☐
	7	The student applies gait belt safely and securely to the patient.	☐	☐	☐
Skill Performance	8	The student correctly performs the **Dynamic Gait Index**:			
		Student correctly explains testing purpose to patient: *(This test is going to assess your gait while performing dynamic tasks).*	☐	☐	☐
		Student correctly performs the test.	☐	☐	☐
		Student provides appropriate guarding techniques. Preferred assistive device is permitted.	☐	☐	☐
		Student determines test score and explains the results: *(0–19 = high risk for falls 20–21 = moderate risk for falls 22–24 = low risk for falls).*	☐	☐	☐
Post-Skill	9	The student washes their hands post–skill performance:			
		Student removes all jewelry from their wrists and hands. Student turns the water to the preferred temperature and wets their hands. Student applies the soap to their hands and washes them with their hands pointed down. Student scrubs for 40–60 seconds and includes palm, between fingers, fingernails, and dorsum of hands. Student rinses hands with hands pointed down. Student dries their hands with a paper towel, uses a paper towel to turn off the water, and then disposes of the paper towel in the trash.	☐	☐	☐
	10	The student verbalizes that they will document their session in the note.	☐	☐	☐
Other	11 ⚑	The student has optimal body mechanics during performance of the skill.	☐	☐	☐
	12 ⚑	The student uses appropriate therapeutic touch.	☐	☐	☐
	13	The student is able to complete the check-off in the time allotted.	☐	☐	☐

⚑ = Critical Safety Element/Professionalism. If a student is unable to complete a flagged step without cueing, they will need to return at another time to redo the check-off. All other steps can be cued.

Communication	14	The student uses language the patient can understand.	☐	☐	☐
	15	The student listens actively to the patient during the session.	☐	☐	☐
	16	The student ensures the patient understands instructions by having the patient teach back or demonstrate.	☐	☐	☐
	17 ⚐	The student demonstrates confidence and provides the patient with clear instruction and cueing.	☐	☐	☐

Peer Name (Printed)		Peer Signature		Date of Peer Review	
Instructor Name (Printed and Signature)	By signing this skills checklist, I am declaring this student competent in the skill described above.			Date of Instructor Review	
NOTES					

⚐ = Critical Safety Element/Professionalism. If a student is unable to complete a flagged step without cueing, they will need to return at another time to redo the check-off. All other steps can be cued.

Sensory Testing

Larson T. *Entry-Level Skill Checklists for*
Physical Therapist Assistant Students (pp 19-21).
© 2023 Taylor & Francis Group.

Student Name: _____

Skill		Sensory Testing: Cranial Nerve Testing			
Source		Lazaro RT, Umphred DA. *Umphred's Neurorehabilitation for the Physical Therapist Assistant.* 3rd ed. SLACK Incorporated; 2021.	**Check When Completed**		
			Self	Peer	Instructor
Student Introduction and Consent	1 ⚑	The student introduces themself to the patient. Must include that they are a **student** PTA and list the school's name.	☐	☐	☐
	2 ⚑	The student verifies the patient's identity. Must use at least 2 patient identifiers (name, date of birth).	☐	☐	☐
	3 ⚑	The student gains consent: • Speaks with the patient about their status (acquires relevant information) • Educates the patient on intended data collection/intervention and goals for the session • Gains permission to perform said data collection/intervention	☐	☐	☐
Student, Patient, and Supply Preparation	4 ⚑	The student gathers supplies and prepares treatment area (cleans equipment, checks for safety hazards, ensures all equipment is functional and appropriate).	☐	☐	☐
	5	The student washes their hands:			
		Student removes all jewelry from their wrists and hands. Student turns the water to the preferred temperature and wets their hands. Student applies the soap to their hands and washes them with their hands pointed down. Student scrubs for 40–60 seconds and includes palm, between fingers, fingernails, and dorsum of hands. Student rinses hands with hands pointed down. Student dries their hands with a paper towel, uses a paper towel to turn off the water, and then disposes of the paper towel in the trash.	☐	☐	☐
	6	The student places the patient in the correct position for support, comfort, and access to body area necessary for data collection/intervention.	☐	☐	☐
Skill Performance	7	The student correctly assesses **Cranial Nerve I**:			
		Student presents familiar, nonirritating odors (citrus, coffee) to each nostril.	☐	☐	☐
		Student asks patient to describe the odor.	☐	☐	☐
	8	The student correctly assesses **Cranial Nerve II**:			
		Student tests patient's ability to perceive objects in different areas of the visual field.	☐	☐	☐
	9	The student correctly assesses **Cranial Nerve III**:			
		Student asks patient to look up, down, inward toward the nose, and combined up and in.	☐	☐	☐
	10	The student correctly assesses **Cranial Nerve IV**:			
		Student asks patient to look down and in concurrently.	☐	☐	☐
	11	The student correctly assesses **Cranial Nerve V**:			
		Student assesses the sensation of the face using a pinprick.	☐	☐	☐
		Student performs manual muscle testing to the muscles of mastication.	☐	☐	☐
	12	The student correctly assesses **Cranial Nerve VI**:			
		Student has patient move their eyes laterally.	☐	☐	☐
	13	The student correctly assesses **Cranial Nerve VII**:			
		Student performs manual muscle testing to the muscles of facial expression.	☐	☐	☐
	14	The student correctly assesses **Cranial Nerve VIII**:			
		Student assesses patient's hearing by rubbing their fingers close to patient's ear and determines if they can hear the sound.	☐	☐	☐

⚑ = Critical Safety Element/Professionalism. If a student is unable to complete a flagged step without cueing, they will need to return at another time to redo the check-off. All other steps can be cued.

	15	The student correctly assesses **Cranial Nerve IX**:			
		Student touches a tongue depressor to the posterior portion of the tongue to determine whether a gag reflex is elicited.	☐	☐	☐
	16	The student correctly assesses **Cranial Nerve X**:			
		Student asks patient to say "ahhhh" and looks for symmetrical elevation of the soft palate.	☐	☐	☐
	17	The student correctly assesses **Cranial Nerve XI**:			
		Student performs manual muscle testing to the trapezius and the sternocleidomastoid muscles.	☐	☐	☐
	18	The student correctly assesses **Cranial Nerve XII**:			
		Student asks patient to protrude their tongue and looks for deviation.	☐	☐	☐
		Student asks patient to push their tongue into their cheek. Student then tests the strength of the tongue by pushing against the cheek from the outside of the cheek.	☐	☐	☐
Post-Skill	19	The student washes their hands post–skill performance:			
		Student removes all jewelry from their wrists and hands. Student turns the water to the preferred temperature and wets their hands. Student applies the soap to their hands and washes them with their hands pointed down. Student scrubs for 40–60 seconds and includes palm, between fingers, fingernails, and dorsum of hands. Student rinses hands with hands pointed down. Student dries their hands with a paper towel, uses a paper towel to turn off the water, and then disposes of the paper towel in the trash.	☐	☐	☐
	20	The student verbalizes that they will document their session in the note.	☐	☐	☐
Other	21 ⚑	The student has optimal body mechanics during performance of the skill.	☐	☐	☐
	22 ⚑	The student uses appropriate therapeutic touch.	☐	☐	☐
	23	The student is able to complete the check-off in the time allotted.	☐	☐	☐
Communication	24	The student uses language the patient can understand.	☐	☐	☐
	25	The student listens actively to the patient during the session.	☐	☐	☐
	26	The student ensures the patient understands instructions by having the patient teach back or demonstrate.	☐	☐	☐
	27 ⚑	The student demonstrates confidence and provides the patient with clear instruction and cueing.	☐	☐	☐

Peer Name (Printed)		**Peer Signature**		**Date of Peer Review**	
Instructor Name (Printed and Signature)	By signing this skills checklist, I am declaring this student competent in the skill described above.			**Date of Instructor Review**	

NOTES	

⚑ = Critical Safety Element/Professionalism. If a student is unable to complete a flagged step without cueing, they will need to return at another time to redo the check-off. All other steps can be cued.

Range of Motion Testing

Larson T. *Entry-Level Skill Checklists for Physical Therapist Assistant Students* (pp 23-47).
© 2023 Taylor & Francis Group.

Student Name: _____

Skill		Range of Motion Testing: Cervical Spine			
Source		Van Ost L, Morogiello J. *Cram Session in Goniometry and Manual Muscle Testing: A Handbook for Students & Clinicians.* 2nd ed. SLACK Incorporated; 2023.	**Check When Completed**		
			Self	Peer	Instructor
Student Introduction and Consent	1 ⚑	The student introduces themself to the patient. Must include that they are a **student** PTA and list the school's name.	☐	☐	☐
	2 ⚑	The student verifies the patient's identity. Must use at least 2 patient identifiers (name, date of birth).	☐	☐	☐
	3 ⚑	The student gains consent: • Speaks with the patient about their status (acquires relevant information) • Educates the patient on intended data collection/intervention and goals for the session • Gains permission to perform said data collection/intervention	☐	☐	☐
Student, Patient, and Supply Preparation	4 ⚑	The student gathers supplies and prepares treatment area (cleans equipment, checks for safety hazards, ensures all equipment is functional and appropriate).	☐	☐	☐
	5	The student washes their hands:			
		Student removes all jewelry from their wrists and hands. Student turns the water to the preferred temperature and wets their hands. Student applies the soap to their hands and washes them with their hands pointed down. Student scrubs for 40–60 seconds and includes palm, between fingers, fingernails, and dorsum of hands. Student rinses hands with hands pointed down. Student dries their hands with a paper towel, uses a paper towel to turn off the water, and then disposes of the paper towel in the trash.	☐	☐	☐
	6	The student places the patient in the correct position for support, comfort, and access to body area necessary for data collection/intervention.	☐	☐	☐
Skill Performance	7	The student correctly measures **Cervical Flexion Active Range of Motion** using goniometer:			
		Student places patient in sitting with the thoracic spine stabilized against a chair.	☐	☐	☐
		Student locates the appropriate landmarks: *(Stationary arm = perpendicular to the floor* *Axis = external auditory meatus* *Movement arm = parallel to the base of the nose).*	☐	☐	☐
		Student asks patient to flex their neck as much as they can.	☐	☐	☐
		Student assesses range of motion and verbalizes findings to instructor.	☐	☐	☐
		Student verbalizes normal range: *(0–45 degrees).*	☐	☐	☐
		Student asks patient if they had any pain during that motion. If yes, student asks patient to rate their pain and documents the results.	☐	☐	☐
	8	The student correctly measures **Cervical Extension Active Range of Motion** using goniometer:			
		Student places patient in sitting with the thoracic spine stabilized against a chair.	☐	☐	☐
		Student locates the appropriate landmarks: *(Stationary arm = perpendicular to the floor* *Axis = external auditory meatus* *Movement arm = parallel to the base of the nose).*	☐	☐	☐
		Student asks patient to extend their neck as much as they can.	☐	☐	☐
		Student assesses range of motion and verbalizes findings to instructor.	☐	☐	☐
		Student verbalizes normal range: *(0–45 degrees).*	☐	☐	☐
		Student asks patient if they had any pain during that motion. If yes, student asks patient to rate their pain and documents the results.	☐	☐	☐

⚑ = Critical Safety Element/Professionalism. If a student is unable to complete a flagged step without cueing, they will need to return at another time to redo the check-off. All other steps can be cued.

	9	The student correctly measures **Cervical Lateral Flexion Active Range of Motion** using goniometer:			
		Student places patient in sitting with the thoracic spine stabilized against a chair.	☐	☐	☐
		Student locates the appropriate landmarks: *(Stationary arm = perpendicular to the floor Axis = center over the spinous process of C7 Movement arm = external occipital protuberance of the occiput).*	☐	☐	☐
		Student asks patient to side bend their neck as much as they can.	☐	☐	☐
		Student assesses range of motion and verbalizes findings to instructor.	☐	☐	☐
		Student verbalizes normal range: *(0–45 degrees).*	☐	☐	☐
		Student asks patient if they had any pain during that motion. If yes, student asks patient to rate their pain and documents the results.	☐	☐	☐
	10	The student correctly measures **Cervical Rotation Active Range of Motion** using goniometer:			
		Student places patient in sitting with the thoracic spine stabilized against a chair.	☐	☐	☐
		Student locates the appropriate landmarks: *(Stationary arm = acromion process of tested side Axis = center of the top of the head Movement arm = tip of the nose).*	☐	☐	☐
		Student asks patient to rotate their neck as much as they can.	☐	☐	☐
		Student assesses range of motion and verbalizes findings to instructor.	☐	☐	☐
		Student verbalizes normal range: *(0–60 degrees).*	☐	☐	☐
		Student asks patient if they had any pain during that motion. If yes, student asks patient to rate their pain and documents the results.	☐	☐	☐
Post-Skill	11	The student washes their hands post–skill performance:			
		Student removes all jewelry from their wrists and hands. Student turns the water to the preferred temperature and wets their hands. Student applies the soap to their hands and washes them with their hands pointed down. Student scrubs for 40–60 seconds and includes palm, between fingers, fingernails, and dorsum of hands. Student rinses hands with hands pointed down. Student dries their hands with a paper towel, uses a paper towel to turn off the water, and then disposes of the paper towel in the trash.	☐	☐	☐
	12	The student verbalizes that they will document their session in the note.	☐	☐	☐
Other	13 ⚑	The student has optimal body mechanics during performance of the skill.	☐	☐	☐
	14 ⚑	The student uses appropriate therapeutic touch.	☐	☐	☐
	15	The student is able to complete the check-off in the time allotted.	☐	☐	☐

⚑ = Critical Safety Element/Professionalism. If a student is unable to complete a flagged step without cueing, they will need to return at another time to redo the check-off. All other steps can be cued.

Communication	16	The student uses language the patient can understand.		☐	☐	☐
	17	The student listens actively to the patient during the session.		☐	☐	☐
	18	The student ensures the patient understands instructions by having the patient teach back or demonstrate.		☐	☐	☐
	19 ⚐	The student demonstrates confidence and provides the patient with clear instruction and cueing.		☐	☐	☐
Peer Name (Printed)			**Peer Signature**		**Date of Peer Review**	
Instructor Name (Printed and Signature)	By signing this skills checklist, I am declaring this student competent in the skill described above.				**Date of Instructor Review**	
NOTES						

⚐ = Critical Safety Element/Professionalism. If a student is unable to complete a flagged step without cueing, they will need to return at another time to redo the check-off. All other steps can be cued.

Student Name: _____

Skill		Range of Motion Testing: Shoulder			
Source		Van Ost L, Morogiello J. *Cram Session in Goniometry and Manual Muscle Testing: A Handbook for Students & Clinicians*. 2nd ed. SLACK Incorporated; 2023.	**Check When Completed**		
			Self	Peer	Instructor
Student Introduction and Consent	1 ⚑	The student introduces themself to the patient. Must include that they are a **student** PTA and list the school's name.	☐	☐	☐
	2 ⚑	The student verifies the patient's identity. Must use at least 2 patient identifiers (name, date of birth).	☐	☐	☐
	3 ⚑	The student gains consent: • Speaks with the patient about their status (acquires relevant information) • Educates the patient on intended data collection/intervention and goals for the session • Gains permission to perform said data collection/intervention	☐	☐	☐
Student, Patient, and Supply Preparation	4 ⚑	The student gathers supplies and prepares treatment area (cleans equipment, checks for safety hazards, ensures all equipment is functional and appropriate).	☐	☐	☐
	5	The student washes their hands:			
		Student removes all jewelry from their wrists and hands. Student turns the water to the preferred temperature and wets their hands. Student applies the soap to their hands and washes them with their hands pointed down. Student scrubs for 40–60 seconds and includes palm, between fingers, fingernails, and dorsum of hands. Student rinses hands with hands pointed down. Student dries their hands with a paper towel, uses a paper towel to turn off the water, and then disposes of the paper towel in the trash.	☐	☐	☐
	6	The student places the patient in the correct position for support, comfort, and access to body area necessary for data collection/intervention.	☐	☐	☐
Skill Performance	7	The student correctly measures **Shoulder Flexion Active Range of Motion** using goniometer:			
		Student places patient in supine with the knees flexed to stabilize the spine.	☐	☐	☐
		Student locates the appropriate landmarks: *(Stationary arm = midaxillary line of the trunk Axis = near the acromion process, through the humeral head Movement arm = lateral epicondyle of humerus).*	☐	☐	☐
		Student asks patient to flex their shoulder as much as they can.	☐	☐	☐
		Student assesses range of motion and verbalizes findings to instructor.	☐	☐	☐
		Student verbalizes normal range: *(0–180 degrees).*	☐	☐	☐
		Student asks patient if they had any pain during that motion. If yes, student asks patient to rate their pain and documents the results.	☐	☐	☐

⚑ = Critical Safety Element/Professionalism. If a student is unable to complete a flagged step without cueing, they will need to return at another time to redo the check-off. All other steps can be cued.

	8	The student correctly measures **Shoulder Abduction Active Range of Motion** using goniometer:			
		Student places patient in supine with the knees flexed to stabilize the spine.	☐	☐	☐
		Student locates the appropriate landmarks: *(Stationary arm = parallel to the midline of the sternum, along the lateral aspect of the trunk* *Axis = near the anterior aspect of the acromion process through the humeral head* *Movement arm = lateral epicondyle of humerus).*	☐	☐	☐
		Student asks patient to abduct their shoulder as much as they can.	☐	☐	☐
		Student assesses range of motion and verbalizes findings to instructor.	☐	☐	☐
		Student verbalizes normal range: *(0–180 degrees).*	☐	☐	☐
		Student asks patient if they had any pain during that motion. If yes, student asks patient to rate their pain and documents the results.	☐	☐	☐
	9	The student correctly measures **Shoulder Internal Rotation Active Range of Motion** using goniometer:			
		Student places patient in supine with shoulder abducted to 90 degrees and elbow flexed to 90 degrees. Student places a towel under the humerus to position it parallel to table.	☐	☐	☐
		Student locates the appropriate landmarks: *(Stationary arm = perpendicular to floor* *Axis = olecranon process of the ulna* *Movement arm = styloid process of the ulna).*	☐	☐	☐
		Student asks patient to internally rotate their shoulder as much as they can.	☐	☐	☐
		Student assesses range of motion and verbalizes findings to instructor.	☐	☐	☐
		Student verbalizes normal range: *(0–75 degrees).*	☐	☐	☐
		Student asks patient if they had any pain during that motion. If yes, student asks patient to rate their pain and documents the results.	☐	☐	☐
	10	The student correctly measures **Shoulder External Rotation Active Range of Motion** using goniometer:			
		Student places patient in supine with shoulder abducted to 90 degrees and elbow flexed to 90 degrees. Student places a towel under the humerus to position it parallel to table.	☐	☐	☐
		Student locates the appropriate landmarks: *(Stationary arm = perpendicular to floor* *Axis = olecranon process of the ulna* *Movement arm = styloid process of the ulna).*	☐	☐	☐
		Student asks patient to externally rotate their shoulder as much as they can.	☐	☐	☐
		Student assesses range of motion and verbalizes findings to instructor.	☐	☐	☐
		Student verbalizes normal range: *(0–90 degrees).*	☐	☐	☐
		Student asks patient if they had any pain during that motion. If yes, student asks patient to rate their pain and documents the results.	☐	☐	☐

☐ = Critical Safety Element/Professionalism. If a student is unable to complete a flagged step without cueing, they will need to return at another time to redo the check-off. All other steps can be cued.

	11	The student correctly measures **Shoulder Extension Active Range of Motion** using goniometer:			
		Student places patient in prone, palm facing ceiling.	☐	☐	☐
		Student locates the appropriate landmarks: *(Stationary arm = midaxillary line of the trunk* *Axis = near the acromion process, through the humeral head* *Movement arm = lateral epicondyle of humerus).*	☐	☐	☐
		Student asks patient to extend their shoulder as much as they can.	☐	☐	☐
		Student assesses range of motion and verbalizes findings to instructor.	☐	☐	☐
		Student verbalizes normal range: *(0–40-60 degrees)*	☐	☐	☐
		Student asks patient if they had any pain during that motion. If yes, student asks patient to rate their pain and documents the results.	☐	☐	☐
Post-Skill	12	The student washes their hands post–skill performance:			
		Student removes all jewelry from their wrists and hands. Student turns the water to the preferred temperature and wets their hands. Student applies the soap to their hands and washes them with their hands pointed down. Student scrubs for 40–60 seconds and includes palm, between fingers, fingernails, and dorsum of hands. Student rinses hands with hands pointed down. Student dries their hands with a paper towel, uses a paper towel to turn off the water, and then disposes of the paper towel in the trash.	☐	☐	☐
	13	The student verbalizes that they will document their session in the note.	☐	☐	☐
Other	14 ⚑	The student has optimal body mechanics during performance of the skill.	☐	☐	☐
	15 ⚑	The student uses appropriate therapeutic touch.	☐	☐	☐
	16	The student is able to complete the check-off in the time allotted.	☐	☐	☐
Communication	17	The student uses language the patient can understand.	☐	☐	☐
	18	The student listens actively to the patient during the session.	☐	☐	☐
	19	The student ensures the patient understands instructions by having the patient teach back or demonstrate.	☐	☐	☐
	20 ⚑	The student demonstrates confidence and provides the patient with clear instruction and cueing.	☐	☐	☐

Peer Name (Printed)		**Peer Signature**		**Date of Peer Review**	
Instructor Name (Printed and Signature)	By signing this skills checklist, I am declaring this student competent in the skill described above.			**Date of Instructor Review**	

NOTES	

⚑ = Critical Safety Element/Professionalism. If a student is unable to complete a flagged step without cueing, they will need to return at another time to redo the check-off. All other steps can be cued.

Student Name: _____

Skill		Range of Motion Testing: Elbow/Forearm			
Source		Van Ost L, Morogiello J. *Cram Session in Goniometry and Manual Muscle Testing: A Handbook for Students & Clinicians*. 2nd ed. SLACK Incorporated; 2023.	**Check When Completed**		
			Self	Peer	Instructor
Student Introduction and Consent	1 ⚐	The student introduces themself to the patient. Must include that they are a **student** PTA and list the school's name.	☐	☐	☐
	2 ⚐	The student verifies the patient's identity. Must use at least 2 patient identifiers (name, date of birth).	☐	☐	☐
	3 ⚐	The student gains consent: • Speaks with the patient about their status (acquires relevant information) • Educates the patient on intended data collection/intervention and goals for the session • Gains permission to perform said data collection/intervention	☐	☐	☐
Student, Patient, and Supply Preparation	4 ⚐	The student gathers supplies and prepares treatment area (cleans equipment, checks for safety hazards, ensures all equipment is functional and appropriate).	☐	☐	☐
	5	The student washes their hands:			
		Student removes all jewelry from their wrists and hands. Student turns the water to the preferred temperature and wets their hands. Student applies the soap to their hands and washes them with their hands pointed down. Student scrubs for 40–60 seconds and includes palm, between fingers, fingernails, and dorsum of hands. Student rinses hands with hands pointed down. Student dries their hands with a paper towel, uses a paper towel to turn off the water, and then disposes of the paper towel in the trash.	☐	☐	☐
	6	The student places the patient in the correct position for support, comfort, and access to body area necessary for data collection/intervention.	☐	☐	☐
Skill Performance	7	The student correctly measures **Elbow Flexion Active Range of Motion** using goniometer:			
		Student places patient in supine with humerus supported on a towel.	☐	☐	☐
		Student locates the appropriate landmarks: *(Stationary arm = lateral midline of the humerus, acromion process Axis = lateral epicondyle of humerus Movement arm = lateral midline of the radius, radial styloid process).*	☐	☐	☐
		Student asks patient to flex their elbow as much as they can.	☐	☐	☐
		Student assesses range of motion and verbalizes findings to instructor.	☐	☐	☐
		Student verbalizes normal range: *(0–145 degrees).*	☐	☐	☐
		Student asks patient if they had any pain during that motion. If yes, student asks patient to rate their pain and documents the results.	☐	☐	☐
	8	The student correctly measures **Elbow Extension Active Range of Motion** using goniometer:			
		Student places patient in supine with humerus supported on a towel.	☐	☐	☐
		Student locates the appropriate landmarks: *(Stationary arm = lateral midline of the humerus, acromion process Axis = lateral epicondyle of humerus Movement arm = lateral midline of the radius, radial styloid process).*	☐	☐	☐
		Student asks patient to extend their elbow as much as they can.	☐	☐	☐
		Student assesses range of motion and verbalizes findings to instructor.	☐	☐	☐
		Student verbalizes normal range: *(145–0 degrees).*	☐	☐	☐
		Student asks patient if they had any pain during that motion. If yes, student asks patient to rate their pain and documents the results.	☐	☐	☐

⚐ = Critical Safety Element/Professionalism. If a student is unable to complete a flagged step without cueing, they will need to return at another time to redo the check-off. All other steps can be cued.

	9	The student correctly measures **Forearm Pronation Active Range of Motion** using goniometer:			
		Student places patient in sitting with shoulder at 0 degrees of abduction, flexion, and extension. The elbow at 90 degrees of flexion and neutral rotation.			
		Student locates the appropriate landmarks: *(Stationary arm = parallel to the anterior midline of humerus Axis = lateral to the ulnar styloid Movement arm = dorsal aspect of wrist, proximal to the styloid process of the ulna and radius).*	☐	☐	☐
		Student asks patient to pronate their forearm as much as they can.	☐	☐	☐
		Student assesses range of motion and verbalizes findings to instructor.	☐	☐	☐
		Student verbalizes normal range: *(0–90 degrees).*	☐	☐	☐
		Student asks patient if they had any pain during that motion. If yes, student asks patient to rate their pain and documents the results.	☐	☐	☐
	10	The student correctly measures **Forearm Supination Active Range of Motion** using goniometer:			
		Student places patient in sitting with shoulder at 0 degrees of abduction, flexion, and extension. The elbow at 90 degrees of flexion and neutral rotation.	☐	☐	☐
		Student locates the appropriate landmarks: *(Stationary arm = parallel to the anterior midline of humerus Axis = medial to the ulnar styloid Movement arm = ventral aspect of wrist, proximal to the styloid process of the ulna and radius).*	☐	☐	☐
		Student asks patient to supinate their forearm as much as they can.	☐	☐	☐
		Student assesses range of motion and verbalizes findings to instructor.	☐	☐	☐
		Student verbalizes normal range: *(0–90 degrees).*	☐	☐	☐
		Student asks patient if they had any pain during that motion. If yes, student asks patient to rate their pain and documents the results.	☐	☐	☐
Post-Skill	11	The student washes their hands post–skill performance:			
		Student removes all jewelry from their wrists and hands. Student turns the water to the preferred temperature and wets their hands. Student applies the soap to their hands and washes them with their hands pointed down. Student scrubs for 40–60 seconds and includes palm, between fingers, fingernails, and dorsum of hands. Student rinses hands with hands pointed down. Student dries their hands with a paper towel, uses a paper towel to turn off the water, and then disposes of the paper towel in the trash.	☐	☐	☐
	12	The student verbalizes that they will document their session in the note.	☐	☐	☐
Other	13 ⚑	The student has optimal body mechanics during performance of the skill.	☐	☐	☐
	14 ⚑	The student uses appropriate therapeutic touch.	☐	☐	☐
	15	The student is able to complete the check-off in the time allotted.	☐	☐	☐

⚑ = Critical Safety Element/Professionalism. If a student is unable to complete a flagged step without cueing, they will need to return at another time to redo the check-off. All other steps can be cued.

Communication	16	The student uses language the patient can understand.	☐	☐	☐
	17	The student listens actively to the patient during the session.	☐	☐	☐
	18	The student ensures the patient understands instructions by having the patient teach back or demonstrate.	☐	☐	☐
	19 ⚑	The student demonstrates confidence and provides the patient with clear instruction and cueing.	☐	☐	☐

Peer Name (Printed)		Peer Signature		Date of Peer Review	
Instructor Name (Printed and Signature)	By signing this skills checklist, I am declaring this student competent in the skill described above.			Date of Instructor Review	

NOTES	

⚑ = Critical Safety Element/Professionalism. If a student is unable to complete a flagged step without cueing, they will need to return at another time to redo the check-off. All other steps can be cued.

Student Name: _____

Skill	Range of Motion Testing: Wrist				
Source	Van Ost L, Morogiello J. *Cram Session in Goniometry and Manual Muscle Testing: A Handbook for Students & Clinicians*. 2nd ed. SLACK Incorporated; 2023.		**Check When Completed**		
			Self	Peer	Instructor
Student Introduction and Consent	1 ⚑	The student introduces themself to the patient. Must include that they are a **student** PTA and list the school's name.	☐	☐	☐
	2 ⚑	The student verifies the patient's identity. Must use at least 2 patient identifiers (name, date of birth).	☐	☐	☐
	3 ⚑	The student gains consent: <ul><li>Speaks with the patient about their status (acquires relevant information)</li><li>Educates the patient on intended data collection/intervention and goals for the session</li><li>Gains permission to perform said data collection/intervention</li></ul>	☐	☐	☐
Student, Patient, and Supply Preparation	4 ⚑	The student gathers supplies and prepares treatment area (cleans equipment, checks for safety hazards, ensures all equipment is functional and appropriate).	☐	☐	☐
	5	The student washes their hands:			
		Student removes all jewelry from their wrists and hands. Student turns the water to the preferred temperature and wets their hands. Student applies the soap to their hands and washes them with their hands pointed down. Student scrubs for 40–60 seconds and includes palm, between fingers, fingernails, and dorsum of hands. Student rinses hands with hands pointed down. Student dries their hands with a paper towel, uses a paper towel to turn off the water, and then disposes of the paper towel in the trash.	☐	☐	☐
	6	The student places the patient in the correct position for support, comfort, and access to body area necessary for data collection/intervention.	☐	☐	☐
Skill Performance	7	The student correctly measures **Wrist Flexion Active Range of Motion** using goniometer:			
		Student places patient in a seated position with forearm pronated and supported on table, wrist hanging off edge of table.	☐	☐	☐
		Student locates the appropriate landmarks: *(Stationary arm = lateral midline of the ulna, olecranon process Axis = lateral aspect of wrist, just distal to the styloid process of the ulna Movement arm = lateral midline of 5th metacarpal).*	☐	☐	☐
		Student asks patient to flex their wrist as much as they can.	☐	☐	☐
		Student assesses range of motion and verbalizes findings to instructor.	☐	☐	☐
		Student verbalizes normal range: *(0–50 degrees).*	☐	☐	☐
		Student asks patient if they had any pain during that motion. If yes, student asks patient to rate their pain and documents the results.	☐	☐	☐

⚑ = Critical Safety Element/Professionalism. If a student is unable to complete a flagged step without cueing, they will need to return at another time to redo the check-off. All other steps can be cued.

	8	The student correctly measures **Wrist Extension Active Range of Motion** using goniometer:			
		Student places patient in a seated position with forearm pronated and supported on table, wrist hanging off edge of table.	☐	☐	☐
		Student locates the appropriate landmarks: *(Stationary arm = lateral midline of the ulna, olecranon process Axis = lateral aspect of wrist, just distal to the styloid process of the ulna Movement arm = lateral midline of 5th metacarpal).*	☐	☐	☐
		Student asks patient to flex their wrist as much as they can.	☐	☐	☐
		Student assesses range of motion and verbalizes findings to instructor.	☐	☐	☐
		Student verbalizes normal range: *(0–70 degrees).*	☐	☐	☐
		Student asks patient if they had any pain during that motion. If yes, student asks patient to rate their pain and documents the results.	☐	☐	☐
	9	The student correctly measures **Wrist Radial Deviation Active Range of Motion** using goniometer:			
		Student places patient in a seated position with shoulder abducted and elbow flexed to 90 degrees, forearm pronated and supported on table.	☐	☐	☐
		Student locates the appropriate landmarks: *(Stationary arm = dorsal midline of the forearm, lateral epicondyle of humerus Axis = capitate Movement arm = midline of the dorsal surface of the 3rd metacarpal).*	☐	☐	☐
		Student asks patient to radial deviate wrist as much as they can.	☐	☐	☐
		Student assesses range of motion and verbalizes findings to instructor.	☐	☐	☐
		Student verbalizes normal range: *(0–25 degrees).*	☐	☐	☐
		Student asks patient if they had any pain during that motion. If yes, student asks patient to rate their pain and documents the results.	☐	☐	☐
	10	The student correctly measures **Wrist Ulnar Deviation Active Range of Motion** using goniometer:			
		Student places patient in a seated position with shoulder abducted and elbow flexed to 90 degrees, forearm pronated and supported on table.	☐	☐	☐
		Student locates the appropriate landmarks: *(Stationary arm = dorsal midline of the forearm, lateral epicondyle of humerus Axis = capitate Movement arm = midline of the dorsal surface of the 3rd metacarpal).*	☐	☐	☐
		Student asks patient to radial deviate wrist as much as they can.	☐	☐	☐
		Student assesses range of motion and verbalizes findings to instructor.	☐	☐	☐
		Student verbalizes normal range: *(0–35 degrees).*	☐	☐	☐
		Student asks patient if they had any pain during that motion. If yes, student asks patient to rate their pain and documents the results.	☐	☐	☐
Post-Skill	11	The student washes their hands post–skill performance:			
		Student removes all jewelry from their wrists and hands. Student turns the water to the preferred temperature and wets their hands. Student applies the soap to their hands and washes them with their hands pointed down. Student scrubs for 40–60 seconds and includes palm, between fingers, fingernails, and dorsum of hands. Student rinses hands with hands pointed down. Student dries their hands with a paper towel, uses a paper towel to turn off the water, and then disposes of the paper towel in the trash.	☐	☐	☐
	12	The student verbalizes that they will document their session in the note.	☐	☐	☐

☐ = Critical Safety Element/Professionalism. If a student is unable to complete a flagged step without cueing, they will need to return at another time to redo the check-off. All other steps can be cued.

	13 ⚑	The student has optimal body mechanics during performance of the skill.	☐	☐	☐
Other	14 ⚑	The student uses appropriate therapeutic touch.	☐	☐	☐
	15	The student is able to complete the check-off in the time allotted.	☐	☐	☐
Communication	16	The student uses language the patient can understand.	☐	☐	☐
	17	The student listens actively to the patient during the session.	☐	☐	☐
	18	The student ensures the patient understands instructions by having the patient teach back or demonstrate.	☐	☐	☐
	19 ⚑	The student demonstrates confidence and provides the patient with clear instruction and cueing.	☐	☐	☐

Peer Name (Printed)		**Peer Signature**		**Date of Peer Review**	
Instructor Name (Printed and Signature)	By signing this skills checklist, I am declaring this student competent in the skill described above.			**Date of Instructor Review**	

NOTES	

⚑ = Critical Safety Element/Professionalism. If a student is unable to complete a flagged step without cueing, they will need to return at another time to redo the check-off. All other steps can be cued.

Student Name: _____

Skill		Range of Motion Testing: Thoracolumbar			
Source		Van Ost L, Morogiello J. *Cram Session in Goniometry and Manual Muscle Testing: A Handbook for Students & Clinicians.* 2nd ed. SLACK Incorporated; 2023.	**Check When Completed**		
			Self	Peer	Instructor
Student Introduction and Consent	1 ⚐	The student introduces themself to the patient. Must include that they are a **student** PTA and list the school's name.	☐	☐	☐
	2 ⚐	The student verifies the patient's identity. Must use at least 2 patient identifiers (name, date of birth).	☐	☐	☐
	3 ⚐	The student gains consent: • Speaks with the patient about their status (acquires relevant information) • Educates the patient on intended data collection/intervention and goals for the session • Gains permission to perform said data collection/intervention	☐	☐	☐
Student, Patient, and Supply Preparation	4 ⚐	The student gathers supplies and prepares treatment area (cleans equipment, checks for safety hazards, ensures all equipment is functional and appropriate).	☐	☐	☐
	5	The student washes their hands:			
		Student removes all jewelry from their wrists and hands. Student turns the water to the preferred temperature and wets their hands. Student applies the soap to their hands and washes them with their hands pointed down. Student scrubs for 40–60 seconds and includes palm, between fingers, fingernails, and dorsum of hands. Student rinses hands with hands pointed down. Student dries their hands with a paper towel, uses a paper towel to turn off the water, and then disposes of the paper towel in the trash.	☐	☐	☐
	6	The student places the patient in the correct position for support, comfort, and access to body area necessary for data collection/intervention.	☐	☐	☐
Skill Performance	7	The student correctly measures **Thoracolumbar Flexion Active Range of Motion** using tape measure:			
		Student places patient in standing.	☐	☐	☐
		Student measures the distance between C7 and S1 in standing.	☐	☐	☐
		Student asks patient to bend forward as far as possible. Observe for any substitutions (knee and/or hip flexion).	☐	☐	☐
		Student measures the distance between C7 and S1 during flexion (and instructs patient to return to neutral when finished).	☐	☐	☐
		Student calculates the difference between the 2 measurements and verbalizes findings to instructor.	☐	☐	☐
		Student verbalizes normal range: *(Approximately 4 inches).*	☐	☐	☐
		Student asks patient if they had any pain during that motion. If yes, student asks patient to rate their pain and documents the results.	☐	☐	☐

⚐ = Critical Safety Element/Professionalism. If a student is unable to complete a flagged step without cueing, they will need to return at another time to redo the check-off. All other steps can be cued.

	8	The student correctly measures **Thoracolumbar Extension Active Range of Motion** using tape measure:			
		Student places patient in standing.	☐	☐	☐
		Student measures the distance between C7 and S1 in standing.	☐	☐	☐
		Student asks patient to bend backward as far as possible. Observe for any substitutions (trunk rotation or lateral bending).	☐	☐	☐
		Student measures the distance between C7 and S1 during extension (and instructs patient to return to neutral when finished).	☐	☐	☐
		Student calculates the difference between the 2 measurements and verbalizes findings to instructor.	☐	☐	☐
		Student verbalizes normal range: *(Approximately 2 inches).*	☐	☐	☐
		Student asks patient if they had any pain during that motion. If yes, student asks patient to rate their pain and documents the results.	☐	☐	☐
	9	The student correctly measures **Thoracolumbar Lateral Flexion Active Range of Motion** using tape measure:			
		Student places patient in standing.	☐	☐	☐
		Student measures the distance between the tip of the middle finger and the floor in standing.	☐	☐	☐
		Student asks patient to laterally flex as far as possible. Observe for any substitutions (trunk rotation, flexion, or extension).	☐	☐	☐
		Student measures the distance between the tip of the middle finger and the floor in lateral flexion (and instructs patient to return to neutral when finished).	☐	☐	☐
		Student calculates the difference between the 2 measurements and verbalizes findings to instructor.	☐	☐	☐
		Student verbalizes normal range: *(Comparison from right to left).*	☐	☐	☐
		Student asks patient if they had any pain during that motion. If yes, student asks patient to rate their pain and documents the results.	☐	☐	☐
	10	The student correctly measures **Thoracolumbar Rotation Active Range of Motion** using goniometer:			
		Student places patient in a seated position with the spine in a neutral position (preferably without a back support).	☐	☐	☐
		Student locates the appropriate landmarks: *(Stationary arm = parallel to an imaginary line between the 2 iliac crests Axis = center of the top of the head Movement arm = parallel to the top of the shoulder, acromion process).*	☐	☐	☐
		Student asks patient to rotate their spine as much as they can.	☐	☐	☐
		Student assesses range of motion and verbalizes findings to instructor.	☐	☐	☐
		Student verbalizes normal range: *(0–45 degrees).*	☐	☐	☐
		Student asks patient if they had any pain during that motion. If yes, student asks patient to rate their pain and documents the results.	☐	☐	☐
Post-Skill	11	The student washes their hands post–skill performance:			
		Student removes all jewelry from their wrists and hands. Student turns the water to the preferred temperature and wets their hands. Student applies the soap to their hands and washes them with their hands pointed down. Student scrubs for 40–60 seconds and includes palm, between fingers, fingernails, and dorsum of hands. Student rinses hands with hands pointed down. Student dries their hands with a paper towel, uses a paper towel to turn off the water, and then disposes of the paper towel in the trash.	☐	☐	☐
	12	The student verbalizes that they will document their session in the note.	☐	☐	☐

⌐ = Critical Safety Element/Professionalism. If a student is unable to complete a flagged step without cueing, they will need to return at another time to redo the check-off. All other steps can be cued.

Other	13 ⚐	The student has optimal body mechanics during performance of the skill.	☐	☐	☐
	14 ⚐	The student uses appropriate therapeutic touch.	☐	☐	☐
	15	The student is able to complete the check-off in the time allotted.	☐	☐	☐
Communication	16	The student uses language the patient can understand.	☐	☐	☐
	17	The student listens actively to the patient during the session.	☐	☐	☐
	18	The student ensures the patient understands instructions by having the patient teach back or demonstrate.	☐	☐	☐
	19 ⚐	The student demonstrates confidence and provides the patient with clear instruction and cueing.	☐	☐	☐

Peer Name (Printed)		Peer Signature		Date of Peer Review	
Instructor Name (Printed and Signature)	By signing this skills checklist, I am declaring this student competent in the skill described above.			Date of Instructor Review	
NOTES					

⚐ = Critical Safety Element/Professionalism. If a student is unable to complete a flagged step without cueing, they will need to return at another time to redo the check-off. All other steps can be cued.

Student Name: _____

Skill		Range of Motion Testing: Hip			
Source		Van Ost L, Morogiello J. *Cram Session in Goniometry and Manual Muscle Testing: A Handbook for Students & Clinicians*. 2nd ed. SLACK Incorporated; 2023.	**Check When Completed**		
			Self	Peer	Instructor
Student Introduction and Consent	1 ⚑	The student introduces themself to the patient. Must include that they are a **student** PTA and list the school's name.	☐	☐	☐
	2 ⚑	The student verifies the patient's identity. Must use at least 2 patient identifiers (name, date of birth).	☐	☐	☐
	3 ⚑	The student gains consent: • Speaks with the patient about their status (acquires relevant information) • Educates the patient on intended data collection/intervention and goals for the session • Gains permission to perform said data collection/intervention	☐	☐	☐
Student, Patient, and Supply Preparation	4 ⚑	The student gathers supplies and prepares treatment area (cleans equipment, checks for safety hazards, ensures all equipment is functional and appropriate).	☐	☐	☐
	5	The student washes their hands:			
		Student removes all jewelry from their wrists and hands. Student turns the water to the preferred temperature and wets their hands. Student applies the soap to their hands and washes them with their hands pointed down. Student scrubs for 40–60 seconds and includes palm, between fingers, fingernails, and dorsum of hands. Student rinses hands with hands pointed down. Student dries their hands with a paper towel, uses a paper towel to turn off the water, and then disposes of the paper towel in the trash.	☐	☐	☐
	6	The student places the patient in the correct position for support, comfort, and access to body area necessary for data collection/intervention.	☐	☐	☐
Skill Performance	7	The student correctly measures **Hip Flexion Active Range of Motion** using goniometer:			
		Student places patient in supine with the hip in a neutral position.	☐	☐	☐
		Student locates the appropriate landmarks: *(Stationary arm = parallel to the lateral midline of pelvis Axis = lateral aspect of hip, greater trochanter of the femur Movement arm = parallel to the lateral midline of the femur, lateral epicondyle of knee).*	☐	☐	☐
		Student asks patient to flex their hip to the chest as much as they can.	☐	☐	☐
		Student assesses range of motion and verbalizes findings to instructor.	☐	☐	☐
		Student verbalizes normal range: *(0–125 degrees).*	☐	☐	☐
		Student asks patient if they had any pain during that motion. If yes, student asks patient to rate their pain and documents the results.	☐	☐	☐

⚑ = Critical Safety Element/Professionalism. If a student is unable to complete a flagged step without cueing, they will need to return at another time to redo the check-off. All other steps can be cued.

	8	The student correctly measures **Hip Abduction Active Range of Motion** using goniometer:			
		Student places patient in supine with the hip in a neutral position.	☐	☐	☐
		Student locates the appropriate landmarks: *(Stationary arm = align with an imaginary line between both anterior and superior iliac spines Axis = anterior aspect of the ipsilateral ASIS Movement arm = anterior midline of the femur, center of patella).*	☐	☐	☐
		Student asks patient to abduct their hip as much as they can.	☐	☐	☐
		Student assesses range of motion and verbalizes findings to instructor.	☐	☐	☐
		Student verbalizes normal range: *(0–45 degrees).*	☐	☐	☐
		Student asks patient if they had any pain during that motion. If yes, student asks patient to rate their pain and documents the results.	☐	☐	☐
	9	The student correctly measures **Hip Adduction Active Range of Motion** using goniometer:			
		Student places patient in supine with the hip in a neutral position.	☐	☐	☐
		Student locates the appropriate landmarks: *(Stationary arm = align with an imaginary line between both anterior and superior iliac spines Axis = anterior aspect of the ipsilateral ASIS Movement arm = anterior midline of the femur, center of patella).*	☐	☐	☐
		Student asks patient to radial deviate wrist as much as they can.	☐	☐	☐
		Student assesses range of motion and verbalizes findings to instructor.	☐	☐	☐
		Student verbalizes normal range: *(0–30 degrees).*	☐	☐	☐
		Student asks patient if they had any pain during that motion. If yes, student asks patient to rate their pain and documents the results.	☐	☐	☐
	10	The student correctly measures **Hip Internal Rotation Active Range of Motion** using goniometer:			
		Student places patient in sitting on edge of bed, hips and knees to 90 degrees.	☐	☐	☐
		Student locates the appropriate landmarks: *(Stationary arm = perpendicular to floor Axis = center over midpatellar surface Movement arm = anterior midline of lower leg, midpoint between the 2 malleoli of the ankle).*	☐	☐	☐
		Student asks patient to internally rotate their hip as much as they can.	☐	☐	☐
		Student assesses range of motion and verbalizes findings to instructor.	☐	☐	☐
		Student verbalizes normal range: *(0–45 degrees).*	☐	☐	☐
		Student asks patient if they had any pain during that motion. If yes, student asks patient to rate their pain and documents the results.	☐	☐	☐

☐ = Critical Safety Element/Professionalism. If a student is unable to complete a flagged step without cueing, they will need to return at another time to redo the check-off. All other steps can be cued.

	11	The student correctly measures **Hip External Rotation Active Range of Motion** using goniometer:			
		Student places patient in sitting on edge of bed, hips and knees to 90 degrees.	☐	☐	☐
		Student locates the appropriate landmarks: *(Stationary arm = perpendicular to floor Axis = center over midpatellar surface Movement arm = anterior midline of lower leg, midpoint between the 2 malleoli of the ankle).*	☐	☐	☐
		Student asks patient to externally rotate their hip as much as they can.	☐	☐	☐
		Student assesses range of motion and verbalizes findings to instructor.	☐	☐	☐
		Student verbalizes normal range: *(0–45 degrees).*	☐	☐	☐
		Student asks patient if they had any pain during that motion. If yes, student asks patient to rate their pain and documents the results.	☐	☐	☐
	12	The student correctly measures **Hip Extension Active Range of Motion** using goniometer:			
		Student places patient in prone with the hip in a neutral position.	☐	☐	☐
		Student locates the appropriate landmarks: *(Stationary arm = parallel to the lateral midline of pelvis Axis = lateral aspect of hip, greater trochanter of the femur Movement arm = parallel to the lateral midline of the femur, lateral epicondyle of knee).*	☐	☐	☐
		Student asks patient to flex their hip to the chest as much as they can.	☐	☐	☐
		Student assesses range of motion and verbalizes findings to instructor.	☐	☐	☐
		Student verbalizes normal range: *(0–15 degrees).*	☐	☐	☐
		Student asks patient if they had any pain during that motion. If yes, student asks patient to rate their pain and documents the results.	☐	☐	☐
Post-Skill	13	The student washes their hands post–skill performance:			
		Student removes all jewelry from their wrists and hands. Student turns the water to the preferred temperature and wets their hands. Student applies the soap to their hands and washes them with their hands pointed down. Student scrubs for 40–60 seconds and includes palm, between fingers, fingernails, and dorsum of hands. Student rinses hands with hands pointed down. Student dries their hands with a paper towel, uses a paper towel to turn off the water, and then disposes of the paper towel in the trash.	☐	☐	☐
	14	The student verbalizes that they will document their session in the note.	☐	☐	☐
Other	15 ⚑	The student has optimal body mechanics during performance of the skill.	☐	☐	☐
	16 ⚑	The student uses appropriate therapeutic touch.	☐	☐	☐
	17	The student is able to complete the check-off in the time allotted.	☐	☐	☐

⚑ = Critical Safety Element/Professionalism. If a student is unable to complete a flagged step without cueing, they will need to return at another time to redo the check-off. All other steps can be cued.

Communication	18	The student uses language the patient can understand.	☐	☐	☐
	19	The student listens actively to the patient during the session.	☐	☐	☐
	20	The student ensures the patient understands instructions by having the patient teach back or demonstrate.	☐	☐	☐
	21 ⚑	The student demonstrates confidence and provides the patient with clear instruction and cueing.	☐	☐	☐

Peer Name (Printed)		Peer Signature		Date of Peer Review	
Instructor Name (Printed and Signature)	By signing this skills checklist, I am declaring this student competent in the skill described above.			Date of Instructor Review	

NOTES	

⚑ = Critical Safety Element/Professionalism. If a student is unable to complete a flagged step without cueing, they will need to return at another time to redo the check-off. All other steps can be cued.

Student Name: _____

Skill		Range of Motion Testing: Knee			
Source		Van Ost L, Morogiello J. *Cram Session in Goniometry and Manual Muscle Testing: A Handbook for Students & Clinicians*. 2nd ed. SLACK Incorporated; 2023.	**Check When Completed**		
			Self	Peer	Instructor
Student Introduction and Consent	1 ⚑	The student introduces themself to the patient. Must include that they are a **student** PTA and list the school's name.	☐	☐	☐
	2 ⚑	The student verifies the patient's identity. Must use at least 2 patient identifiers (name, date of birth).	☐	☐	☐
	3 ⚑	The student gains consent: • Speaks with the patient about their status (acquires relevant information) • Educates the patient on intended data collection/intervention and goals for the session • Gains permission to perform said data collection/intervention	☐	☐	☐
Student, Patient, and Supply Preparation	4 ⚑	The student gathers supplies and prepares treatment area (cleans equipment, checks for safety hazards, ensures all equipment is functional and appropriate).	☐	☐	☐
	5	The student washes their hands:			
		Student removes all jewelry from their wrists and hands. Student turns the water to the preferred temperature and wets their hands. Student applies the soap to their hands and washes them with their hands pointed down. Student scrubs for 40–60 seconds and includes palm, between fingers, fingernails, and dorsum of hands. Student rinses hands with hands pointed down. Student dries their hands with a paper towel, uses a paper towel to turn off the water, and then disposes of the paper towel in the trash.	☐	☐	☐
	6	The student places the patient in the correct position for support, comfort, and access to body area necessary for data collection/intervention.	☐	☐	☐
Skill Performance	7	The student correctly measures **Knee Flexion Active Range of Motion** using goniometer:			
		Student places patient in supine.	☐	☐	☐
		Student locates the appropriate landmarks: *(Stationary arm = lateral midline of femur to greater trochanter Axis = lateral epicondyle of the knee Movement arm = lateral midline of fibula to lateral malleolus).*	☐	☐	☐
		Student asks patient to flex their knee as much as they can.	☐	☐	☐
		Student assesses range of motion and verbalizes findings to instructor.	☐	☐	☐
		Student verbalizes normal range: *(0–135 degrees).*	☐	☐	☐
		Student asks patient if they had any pain during that motion. If yes, student asks patient to rate their pain and documents the results.	☐	☐	☐

⚑ = Critical Safety Element/Professionalism. If a student is unable to complete a flagged step without cueing, they will need to return at another time to redo the check-off. All other steps can be cued.

	8	The student correctly measures **Knee Extension Active Range of Motion** using goniometer:			
Post-Skill		Student places patient in prone with hip in neutral. A folded towel should be placed under the anterior thigh. Patient is in maximally knee flexed position.	☐	☐	☐
		Student locates the appropriate landmarks: *(Stationary arm = lateral midline of femur to greater trochanter Axis = lateral epicondyle of the knee Movement arm = lateral midline of fibula to lateral malleolus).*	☐	☐	☐
		Student asks patient to extend their knee as much as they can.	☐	☐	☐
		Student assesses range of motion and verbalizes findings to instructor.	☐	☐	☐
		Student verbalizes normal range: *(120–0 degrees).*	☐	☐	☐
		Student asks patient if they had any pain during that motion. If yes, student asks patient to rate their pain and documents the results.	☐	☐	☐
	9	The student washes their hands post–skill performance:			
		Student removes all jewelry from their wrists and hands. Student turns the water to the preferred temperature and wets their hands. Student applies the soap to their hands and washes them with their hands pointed down. Student scrubs for 40–60 seconds and includes palm, between fingers, fingernails, and dorsum of hands. Student rinses hands with hands pointed down. Student dries their hands with a paper towel, uses a paper towel to turn off the water, and then disposes of the paper towel in the trash.	☐	☐	☐
	10	The student verbalizes that they will document their session in the note.	☐	☐	☐
Other	11 ⚑	The student has optimal body mechanics during performance of the skill.	☐	☐	☐
	12 ⚑	The student uses appropriate therapeutic touch.	☐	☐	☐
	13	The student is able to complete the check-off in the time allotted.	☐	☐	☐
Communication	14	The student uses language the patient can understand.	☐	☐	☐
	15	The student listens actively to the patient during the session.	☐	☐	☐
	16	The student ensures the patient understands instructions by having the patient teach back or demonstrate.	☐	☐	☐
	17 ⚑	The student demonstrates confidence and provides the patient with clear instruction and cueing.	☐	☐	☐

Peer Name (Printed)		Peer Signature		Date of Peer Review	
Instructor Name (Printed and Signature)	By signing this skills checklist, I am declaring this student competent in the skill described above.			Date of Instructor Review	

NOTES	

⚑ = Critical Safety Element/Professionalism. If a student is unable to complete a flagged step without cueing, they will need to return at another time to redo the check-off. All other steps can be cued.

Student Name: _____

Skill		Range of Motion Testing: Ankle			
Source		Van Ost L, Morogiello J. *Cram Session in Goniometry and Manual Muscle Testing:* *A Handbook for Students & Clinicians*. 2nd ed. SLACK Incorporated; 2023.	**Check When Completed**		
			Self	Peer	Instructor
Student Introduction and Consent	1 ⚑	The student introduces themself to the patient. Must include that they are a **student** PTA and list the school's name.	☐	☐	☐
	2 ⚑	The student verifies the patient's identity. Must use at least 2 patient identifiers (name, date of birth).	☐	☐	☐
	3 ⚑	The student gains consent: • Speaks with the patient about their status (acquires relevant information) • Educates the patient on intended data collection/intervention and goals for the session • Gains permission to perform said data collection/intervention	☐	☐	☐
Student, Patient, and Supply Preparation	4 ⚑	The student gathers supplies and prepares treatment area (cleans equipment, checks for safety hazards, ensures all equipment is functional and appropriate).	☐	☐	☐
	5	The student washes their hands:			
		Student removes all jewelry from their wrists and hands. Student turns the water to the preferred temperature and wets their hands. Student applies the soap to their hands and washes them with their hands pointed down. Student scrubs for 40–60 seconds and includes palm, between fingers, fingernails, and dorsum of hands. Student rinses hands with hands pointed down. Student dries their hands with a paper towel, uses a paper towel to turn off the water, and then disposes of the paper towel in the trash.	☐	☐	☐
	6	The student places the patient in the correct position for support, comfort, and access to body area necessary for data collection/intervention.	☐	☐	☐
Skill Performance	7	The student correctly measures **Ankle Dorsiflexion Active Range of Motion** using goniometer:			
		Student places patient in sitting or supine with the knee flexed to at least 30 degrees, the foot in midway between inversion and eversion.	☐	☐	☐
		Student locates the appropriate landmarks: *(Stationary arm = lateral midline of fibula, fibular head* *Axis = lateral aspect of the lateral malleolus* *Movement arm = parallel to 5th metatarsal).*	☐	☐	☐
		Student asks patient to dorsiflex their ankle as much as they can.	☐	☐	☐
		Student assesses range of motion and verbalizes findings to instructor.	☐	☐	☐
		Student verbalizes normal range: *(0–20 degrees).*	☐	☐	☐
		Student asks patient if they had any pain during that motion. If yes, student asks patient to rate their pain and documents the results.	☐	☐	☐

⚑ = Critical Safety Element/Professionalism. If a student is unable to complete a flagged step without cueing, they will need to return at another time to redo the check-off. All other steps can be cued.

	8	The student correctly measures **Ankle Plantarflexion Active Range of Motion** using goniometer:			
		Student places patient in sitting or supine with the knee flexed to at least 30 degrees, the foot in midway between inversion and eversion.	☐	☐	☐
		Student locates the appropriate landmarks: *(Stationary arm = lateral midline of fibula to fibular head Axis = lateral aspect of the lateral malleolus Movement arm = parallel to 5th metatarsal).*	☐	☐	☐
		Student asks patient to plantarflex their ankle as much as they can.	☐	☐	☐
		Student assesses range of motion and verbalizes findings to instructor.	☐	☐	☐
		Student verbalizes normal range: *(0–45 degrees).*	☐	☐	☐
		Student asks patient if they had any pain during that motion. If yes, student asks patient to rate their pain and documents the results.	☐	☐	☐
	9	The student correctly measures **Midtarsal Inversion Active Range of Motion** using goniometer:			
		Student places patient in a seated position on edge of table with knee flexed to 90 degrees.	☐	☐	☐
		Student locates the appropriate landmarks: *(Stationary arm = anterior midline of tibia to tibial tuberosity Axis = center over the anterior aspect of ankle midway between the malleoli Movement arm = dorsal aspect of the 2nd metatarsal).*	☐	☐	☐
		Student asks patient to invert their ankle as much as they can.	☐	☐	☐
		Student assesses range of motion and verbalizes findings to instructor.	☐	☐	☐
		Student verbalizes normal range: *(0–30 degrees).*	☐	☐	☐
		Student asks patient if they had any pain during that motion. If yes, student asks patient to rate their pain and documents the results.	☐	☐	☐
	10	The student correctly measures **Midtarsal Eversion Active Range of Motion** using goniometer:			
		Student places patient in a seated position on edge of table with knee flexed to 90 degrees.	☐	☐	☐
		Student locates the appropriate landmarks: *(Stationary arm = anterior midline of tibia to tibial tuberosity Axis = center over the anterior aspect of ankle midway between the malleoli Movement arm = dorsal aspect of the 2nd metatarsal).*	☐	☐	☐
		Student asks patient to evert their ankle as much as they can.	☐	☐	☐
		Student assesses range of motion and verbalizes findings to instructor.	☐	☐	☐
		Student verbalizes normal range: *(0–25 degrees).*	☐	☐	☐
		Student asks patient if they had any pain during that motion. If yes, student asks patient to rate their pain and documents the results.	☐	☐	☐
Post-Skill	11	The student washes their hands post–skill performance:			
		Student removes all jewelry from their wrists and hands. Student turns the water to the preferred temperature and wets their hands. Student applies the soap to their hands and washes them with their hands pointed down. Student scrubs for 40–60 seconds and includes palm, between fingers, fingernails, and dorsum of hands. Student rinses hands with hands pointed down. Student dries their hands with a paper towel, uses a paper towel to turn off the water, and then disposes of the paper towel in the trash.	☐	☐	☐
	12	The student verbalizes that they will document their session in the note.	☐	☐	☐

☐ = Critical Safety Element/Professionalism. If a student is unable to complete a flagged step without cueing, they will need to return at another time to redo the check-off. All other steps can be cued.

Other	13 ⚑	The student has optimal body mechanics during performance of the skill.		☐	☐	☐
	14 ⚑	The student uses appropriate therapeutic touch.		☐	☐	☐
	15	The student is able to complete the check-off in the time allotted.		☐	☐	☐
Communication	16	The student uses language the patient can understand.		☐	☐	☐
	17	The student listens actively to the patient during the session.		☐	☐	☐
	18	The student ensures the patient understands instructions by having the patient teach back or demonstrate.		☐	☐	☐
	19 ⚑	The student demonstrates confidence and provides the patient with clear instruction and cueing.		☐	☐	☐
Peer Name (Printed)			**Peer Signature**		**Date of Peer Review**	
Instructor Name (Printed and Signature)	By signing this skills checklist, I am declaring this student competent in the skill described above.				**Date of Instructor Review**	
NOTES						

⚑ = Critical Safety Element/Professionalism. If a student is unable to complete a flagged step without cueing, they will need to return at another time to redo the check-off. All other steps can be cued.

Chapter 5
Manual Muscle Testing

Larson T. *Entry-Level Skill Checklists for*
Physical Therapist Assistant Students (pp 49-87).
© 2023 Taylor & Francis Group.

Key to Manual Muscle Testing Grades

Muscle Activity	Grade (0–5)
No contraction felt in muscle	0
Tendon is prominent and muscle contraction is palpable, no visible movement of tested body part	1
Moves through complete range of motion in a gravity minimized position	2
Holds test position without resistance	3
Holds test position against moderate resistance	4
Holds test position against strong resistance	5

= Critical Safety Element/Professionalism. If a student is unable to complete a flagged step without cueing, they will need to return at another time to redo the check-off. All other steps can be cued.

Student Name: _____

Skill		Manual Muscle Testing: Cervical Spine			
Source		Van Ost L, Morogiello J. *Cram Session in Goniometry and Manual Muscle Testing: A Handbook for Students & Clinicians.* 2nd ed. SLACK Incorporated; 2023.	Check When Completed		
			Self	Peer	Instructor
Student Introduction and Consent	1 ⚑	The student introduces themself to the patient. Must include that they are a **student** PTA and list the school's name.	☐	☐	☐
	2 ⚑	The student verifies the patient's identity. Must use at least 2 patient identifiers (name, date of birth).	☐	☐	☐
	3 ⚑	The student gains consent: • Speaks with the patient about their status (acquires relevant information) • Educates the patient on intended data collection/intervention and goals for the session • Gains permission to perform said data collection/intervention	☐	☐	☐
Student, Patient, and Supply Preparation	4 ⚑	The student gathers supplies and prepares treatment area (cleans equipment, checks for safety hazards, ensures all equipment is functional and appropriate).	☐	☐	☐
	5	The student washes their hands:			
		Student removes all jewelry from their wrists and hands. Student turns the water to the preferred temperature and wets their hands. Student applies the soap to their hands and washes them with their hands pointed down. Student scrubs for 40–60 seconds and includes palm, between fingers, fingernails, and dorsum of hands. Student rinses hands with hands pointed down. Student dries their hands with a paper towel, uses a paper towel to turn off the water, and then disposes of the paper towel in the trash.	☐	☐	☐
	6	The student places the patient in the correct position for support, comfort, and access to body area necessary for data collection/intervention.	☐	☐	☐
Skill Performance	7	The student correctly measures **Cervical Flexion MMT (against gravity):**			
		Student verbalizes the primary muscle they are assessing: *(Sternocleidomastoid).*	☐	☐	☐
		Student places patient in a supine position.	☐	☐	☐
		Student instructs patient to flex their neck through their full range of motion to ensure full active range of motion.	☐	☐	☐
		Student instructs patient to repeat that motion and then hold in mid-range (20–30 degrees of flexion).	☐	☐	☐
		Student applies stabilization to the thorax.	☐	☐	☐
		Student instructs patient to: *(Hold your neck in this position and do not let me push it down).*	☐	☐	☐
		Student applies moderate resistance to the anterior forehead.	☐	☐	☐
		Student grades the strength of the neck flexors and verbalizes it to instructor.	☐	☐	☐
		Student asks patient if they had any pain during that motion. If yes, student asks patient to rate their pain and documents the results.	☐	☐	☐
	8	The student correctly measures **Cervical Flexion MMT (gravity minimized):**			
		Student places patient in sidelying position with the head supported on a smooth surface.	☐	☐	☐
		Student instructs patient to flex the neck through the range of motion. If no motion occurs at the joint, student palpates the muscle tendons to determine if there is a contraction.	☐	☐	☐
		Student grades the strength of the neck flexors and verbalizes it to instructor.	☐	☐	☐
		Student asks patient if they had any pain during that motion. If yes, student asks patient to rate their pain and documents the results.	☐	☐	☐

⚑ = Critical Safety Element/Professionalism. If a student is unable to complete a flagged step without cueing, they will need to return at another time to redo the check-off. All other steps can be cued.

	9	The student correctly measures **Cervical Extension MMT (against gravity):**			
		Student verbalizes the primary muscles they are assessing: *(Splenius capitis, semispinalis capitis, cervicis muscles).*	☐	☐	☐
		Student places patient in a prone position.	☐	☐	☐
		Student instructs patient to extend their neck through their full range of motion to ensure full active range of motion.	☐	☐	☐
		Student instructs patient to repeat that motion and then hold in mid-range (20–30 degrees of flexion).	☐	☐	☐
		Student applies stabilization to the upper thoracic area.	☐	☐	☐
		Student instructs patient to: *(Hold your neck in this position and do not let me push it down).*	☐	☐	☐
		Student applies moderate resistance to the occiput.	☐	☐	☐
		Student grades the strength of the neck extensors and verbalizes it to instructor.	☐	☐	☐
		Student asks patient if they had any pain during that motion. If yes, student asks patient to rate their pain and documents the results.	☐	☐	☐
	10	The student correctly measures **Cervical Extension MMT (gravity minimized):**			
		Student places patient in sidelying position with the head supported on a smooth surface.	☐	☐	☐
		Student instructs patient to extend the neck through the range of motion. If no motion occurs at the joint, student palpates the muscle tendons to determine if there is a contraction.	☐	☐	☐
		Student grades the strength of the neck extensors and verbalizes it to instructor.	☐	☐	☐
		Student asks patient if they had any pain during that motion. If yes, student asks patient to rate their pain and documents the results.	☐	☐	☐
Post-Skill	11	The student washes their hands post–skill performance:			
		Student removes all jewelry from their wrists and hands. Student turns the water to the preferred temperature and wets their hands. Student applies the soap to their hands and washes them with their hands pointed down. Student scrubs for 40–60 seconds and includes palm, between fingers, fingernails, and dorsum of hands. Student rinses hands with hands pointed down. Student dries their hands with a paper towel, uses a paper towel to turn off the water, and then disposes of the paper towel in the trash.	☐	☐	☐
	12	The student verbalizes that they will document their session in the note.	☐	☐	☐
Other	13 ⚐	The student has optimal body mechanics during performance of the skill.	☐	☐	☐
	14 ⚐	The student uses appropriate therapeutic touch.	☐	☐	☐
	15	The student is able to complete the check-off in the time allotted.	☐	☐	☐

⚐ = Critical Safety Element/Professionalism. If a student is unable to complete a flagged step without cueing, they will need to return at another time to redo the check-off. All other steps can be cued.

Communication	16	The student uses language the patient can understand.	☐	☐	☐
	17	The student listens actively to the patient during the session.	☐	☐	☐
	18	The student ensures the patient understands instructions by having the patient teach back or demonstrate.	☐	☐	☐
	19 ⚑	The student demonstrates confidence and provides the patient with clear instruction and cueing.	☐	☐	☐

Peer Name (Printed)		**Peer Signature**		**Date of Peer Review**	
Instructor Name (Printed and Signature)	By signing this skills checklist, I am declaring this student competent in the skill described above.			**Date of Instructor Review**	

NOTES	

⚑ = Critical Safety Element/Professionalism. If a student is unable to complete a flagged step without cueing, they will need to return at another time to redo the check-off. All other steps can be cued.

Student Name: _____

Skill	Manual Muscle Testing: Scapula			
Source	Van Ost L, Morogiello J. *Cram Session in Goniometry and Manual Muscle Testing: A Handbook for Students & Clinicians.* 2nd ed. SLACK Incorporated; 2023.	**Check When Completed**		
		Self	Peer	Instructor
Student Introduction and Consent	1 ⚑ The student introduces themself to the patient. Must include that they are a **student** PTA and list the school's name.	☐	☐	☐
	2 ⚑ The student verifies the patient's identity. Must use at least 2 patient identifiers (name, date of birth).	☐	☐	☐
	3 ⚑ The student gains consent: • Speaks with the patient about their status (acquires relevant information) • Educates the patient on intended data collection/intervention and goals for the session • Gains permission to perform said data collection/intervention	☐	☐	☐
Student, Patient, and Supply Preparation	4 ⚑ The student gathers supplies and prepares treatment area (cleans equipment, checks for safety hazards, ensures all equipment is functional and appropriate).	☐	☐	☐
	5 The student washes their hands:			
	Student removes all jewelry from their wrists and hands. Student turns the water to the preferred temperature and wets their hands. Student applies the soap to their hands and washes them with their hands pointed down. Student scrubs for 40–60 seconds and includes palm, between fingers, fingernails, and dorsum of hands. Student rinses hands with hands pointed down. Student dries their hands with a paper towel, uses a paper towel to turn off the water, and then disposes of the paper towel in the trash.	☐	☐	☐
	6 The student places the patient in the correct position for support, comfort, and access to body area necessary for data collection/intervention.	☐	☐	☐
Skill Performance	7 The student correctly measures **Scapula Abduction/Upward Rotation MMT (against gravity)**:			
	Student verbalizes the primary muscle they are assessing: *(Serratus anterior).*	☐	☐	☐
	Student places patient in a supine position with the shoulder flexed to 90 degrees and the elbow in extension.	☐	☐	☐
	Student instructs patient to abduct/upward rotate their scapula (punch ceiling) through their full range of motion to ensure full active range of motion.	☐	☐	☐
	Student instructs patient to repeat that motion and then hold their arm in mid-range.	☐	☐	☐
	Student instructs patient to: *(Hold your arm in this position and do not let me push it down).*	☐	☐	☐
	Student applies moderate resistance in a downward/inward direction by grasping the forearm and elbow.	☐	☐	☐
	Student grades the strength of the serratus anterior and verbalizes it to instructor.	☐	☐	☐
	Student asks patient if they had any pain during that motion. If yes, student asks patient to rate their pain and documents the results.	☐	☐	☐
	8 The student correctly measures **Scapula Abduction/Upward Rotation MMT (gravity minimized)**:			
	Student places patient in sitting with the upper arm resting on a table in 90 degrees of shoulder flexion and with the elbow extended.	☐	☐	☐
	Student instructs patient to abduct/upward rotate their scapula (punch forward) through the range of motion. If no motion occurs at the joint, student palpates the muscle tendons to determine if there is a contraction.	☐	☐	☐
	Student grades the strength of the serratus anterior and verbalizes it to instructor.	☐	☐	☐
	Student asks patient if they had any pain during that motion. If yes, student asks patient to rate their pain and documents the results.	☐	☐	☐

⚑ = Critical Safety Element/Professionalism. If a student is unable to complete a flagged step without cueing, they will need to return at another time to redo the check-off. All other steps can be cued.

9	The student correctly measures **Scapula Adduction/Downward Rotation MMT (against gravity)**:				
	Student verbalizes the primary muscles they are assessing: *(Rhomboid major, rhomboid minor).*	☐	☐	☐
	Student places patient in a prone position with the tested upper extremity behind the back with the hand resting on the lumbar spine. The head is rotated to the opposite side.	☐	☐	☐
	Student instructs patient to adduct/downward rotate their scapula (lift hand off the back) through their full range of motion to ensure full active range of motion.	☐	☐	☐
	Student instructs patient to repeat that motion and then hold their arm in mid-range.	☐	☐	☐
	Student applies stabilization to the thorax on the opposite side.	☐	☐	☐
	Student instructs patient to: *(Hold your arm in this position and do not let me push it down).*	☐	☐	☐
	Student applies moderate resistance above the elbow in a down and out direction, pushing the scapula into abduction and upward rotation.	☐	☐	☐
	Student grades the strength of the rhomboids and verbalizes it to instructor.	☐	☐	☐
	Student asks patient if they had any pain during that motion. If yes, student asks patient to rate their pain and documents the results.	☐	☐	☐
10	The student correctly measures **Scapula Adduction/Downward Rotation MMT (gravity minimized)**:				
	Student places patient in seated position with the tested arm internally rotated and adducted behind the lumbar spine.	☐	☐	☐
	Student instructs patient to adduct/downward rotate their scapula (lift hand off the back) through the range of motion. If no motion occurs at the joint, student palpates the muscle tendons to determine if there is a contraction.	☐	☐	☐
	Student grades the strength of the rhomboids and verbalizes it to instructor.	☐	☐	☐
	Student asks patient if they had any pain during that motion. If yes, student asks patient to rate their pain and documents the results.	☐	☐	☐
11	The student correctly measures **Scapula Elevation MMT (against gravity)**:				
	Student verbalizes the primary muscles they are assessing: *(Upper trapezius, levator scapulae).*	☐	☐	☐
	Student places patient in a seated position, with the arms hanging by the sides.	☐	☐	☐
	Student instructs patient to elevate their scapula through their full range of motion to ensure full active range of motion.	☐	☐	☐
	Student instructs patient to repeat that motion and then hold the position.	☐	☐	☐
	Student instructs patient to: *(Hold this position and do not let me push you down).*	☐	☐	☐
	Student applies moderate resistance symmetrically in a downward direction on top of the shoulders.	☐	☐	☐
	Student grades the strength of the scapular elevators and verbalizes it to instructor.	☐	☐	☐
	Student asks patient if they had any pain during that motion. If yes, student asks patient to rate their pain and documents the results.	☐	☐	☐
12	The student correctly measures **Scapula Elevation MMT (gravity minimized)**:				
	Student places patient in supine or prone with the arms resting by the sides.	☐	☐	☐
	Student instructs patient to elevate their scapula through the range of motion. If no motion occurs at the joint, student palpates the muscle tendons to determine if there is a contraction.	☐	☐	☐
	Student grades the strength of the scapular elevators and verbalizes it to instructor.	☐	☐	☐
	Student asks patient if they had any pain during that motion. If yes, student asks patient to rate their pain and documents the results.	☐	☐	☐

☐ = Critical Safety Element/Professionalism. If a student is unable to complete a flagged step without cueing, they will need to return at another time to redo the check-off. All other steps can be cued.

	13	The student correctly measures **Scapula Adduction MMT (against gravity):**			
		Student verbalizes the primary muscles they are assessing: *(Middle trapezius, rhomboid major, rhomboid minor).*	☐	☐	☐
		Student places patient in a prone position with the shoulder in 90 degrees of abduction with the elbow flexed to 90 degrees, the forearm hanging freely off the table.	☐	☐	☐
		Student instructs patient to adduct their scapula through their full range of motion to ensure full active range of motion.	☐	☐	☐
		Student instructs patient to repeat that motion and then hold.	☐	☐	☐
		Student applies stabilization to the contralateral thorax.	☐	☐	☐
		Student instructs patient to: *(Hold your arm in this position and do not let me push it down).*	☐	☐	☐
		Student applies moderate resistance just proximal to the elbow toward the floor.	☐	☐	☐
		Student grades the strength of the scapular adductors and verbalizes it to instructor.	☐	☐	☐
		Student asks patient if they had any pain during that motion. If yes, student asks patient to rate their pain and documents the results.	☐	☐	☐
	14	The student correctly measures **Scapula Adduction MMT (gravity minimized):**			
		Student places patient in sitting with the arm supported on a table in 90 degrees of shoulder abduction and elbow flexion.	☐	☐	☐
		Student instructs patient to adduct the scapula through the range of motion. If no motion occurs at the joint, student palpates the muscle tendons to determine if there is a contraction.	☐	☐	☐
		Student grades the strength of the shoulder scapular adductors and verbalizes it to instructor.	☐	☐	☐
		Student asks patient if they had any pain during that motion. If yes, student asks patient to rate their pain and documents the results.	☐	☐	☐
	15	The student correctly measures **Scapula Depression/Adduction MMT (against gravity):**			
		Student verbalizes the primary muscle they are assessing: *(Lower trapezius).*	☐	☐	☐
		Student places patient in a prone position with the head rotated to the same side as the tested shoulder in approximately 130 degrees of abduction and the elbow in extension.	☐	☐	☐
		Student instructs patient to depress/adduct their scapula (lift arm off the table) through their full range of motion to ensure full active range of motion.	☐	☐	☐
		Student instructs patient to repeat that motion and then hold.	☐	☐	☐
		Student applies stabilization to the contralateral thorax.	☐	☐	☐
		Student instructs patient to: *(Hold your arm in this position and do not let me push it down).*	☐	☐	☐
		Student applies moderate resistance just proximal to the elbow joint, directed to the floor.	☐	☐	☐
		Student grades the strength of the lower trapezius and verbalizes it to instructor.	☐	☐	☐
		Student asks patient if they had any pain during that motion. If yes, student asks patient to rate their pain and documents the results.	☐	☐	☐

⚑ = Critical Safety Element/Professionalism. If a student is unable to complete a flagged step without cueing, they will need to return at another time to redo the check-off. All other steps can be cued.

	16	The student correctly measures **Scapula Depression/Adduction MMT (gravity minimized)**:			
		Student places patient in prone with the head rotated to the same side as the tested shoulder in approximately 130 degrees of abduction.	☐	☐	☐
		Student instructs patient to depress/adduct their scapula (lift arm off the table) through the range of motion. If no motion occurs at the joint, student palpates the muscle tendons to determine if there is a contraction.	☐	☐	☐
		Student grades the strength of the lower trapezius and verbalizes it to instructor.	☐	☐	☐
		Student asks patient if they had any pain during that motion. If yes, student asks patient to rate their pain and documents the results.	☐	☐	☐
Post-Skill	17	The student washes their hands post–skill performance:			
		Student removes all jewelry from their wrists and hands. Student turns the water to the preferred temperature and wets their hands. Student applies the soap to their hands and washes them with their hands pointed down. Student scrubs for 40–60 seconds and includes palm, between fingers, fingernails, and dorsum of hands. Student rinses hands with hands pointed down. Student dries their hands with a paper towel, uses a paper towel to turn off the water, and then disposes of the paper towel in the trash.	☐	☐	☐
	18	The student verbalizes that they will document their session in the note.	☐	☐	☐
Other	19 ⚑	The student has optimal body mechanics during performance of the skill.	☐	☐	☐
	20 ⚑	The student uses appropriate therapeutic touch.	☐	☐	☐
	21	The student is able to complete the check-off in the time allotted.	☐	☐	☐
Communication	22	The student uses language the patient can understand.	☐	☐	☐
	23	The student listens actively to the patient during the session.	☐	☐	☐
	24	The student ensures the patient understands instructions by having the patient teach back or demonstrate.	☐	☐	☐
	25 ⚑	The student demonstrates confidence and provides the patient with clear instruction and cueing.	☐	☐	☐
Peer Name (Printed)			**Peer Signature**			**Date of Peer Review**	
Instructor Name (Printed and Signature)	By signing this skills checklist, I am declaring this student competent in the skill described above.			**Date of Instructor Review**	
NOTES					

⚑ = Critical Safety Element/Professionalism. If a student is unable to complete a flagged step without cueing, they will need to return at another time to redo the check-off. All other steps can be cued.

Student Name: _____

Skill		Manual Muscle Testing: Shoulder			
Source		Van Ost L, Morogiello J. *Cram Session in Goniometry and Manual Muscle Testing: A Handbook for Students & Clinicians*. 2nd ed. SLACK Incorporated; 2023.	Check When Completed		
			Self	Peer	Instructor
Student Introduction and Consent	1 ⚑	The student introduces themself to the patient. Must include that they are a **student** PTA and list the school's name.	☐	☐	☐
	2 ⚑	The student verifies the patient's identity. Must use at least 2 patient identifiers (name, date of birth).	☐	☐	☐
	3 ⚑	The student gains consent: • Speaks with the patient about their status (acquires relevant information) • Educates the patient on intended data collection/intervention and goals for the session • Gains permission to perform said data collection/intervention	☐	☐	☐
Student, Patient, and Supply Preparation	4 ⚑	The student gathers supplies and prepares treatment area (cleans equipment, checks for safety hazards, ensures all equipment is functional and appropriate).	☐	☐	☐
	5	The student washes their hands:			
		Student removes all jewelry from their wrists and hands. Student turns the water to the preferred temperature and wets their hands. Student applies the soap to their hands and washes them with their hands pointed down. Student scrubs for 40–60 seconds and includes palm, between fingers, fingernails, and dorsum of hands. Student rinses hands with hands pointed down. Student dries their hands with a paper towel, uses a paper towel to turn off the water, and then disposes of the paper towel in the trash.	☐	☐	☐
	6	The student places the patient in the correct position for support, comfort, and access to body area necessary for data collection/intervention.	☐	☐	☐
Skill Performance	7	The student correctly measures **Shoulder Flexion MMT (against gravity)**:			
		Student verbalizes the primary muscles they are assessing: *(Anterior deltoid, coracobrachialis).*	☐	☐	☐
		Student places patient in a seated position with legs off the edge of the bed.	☐	☐	☐
		Student instructs patient to flex their shoulder through their full range of motion to ensure full active range of motion.	☐	☐	☐
		Student instructs patient to repeat that motion and then hold their arm in mid-range (90 degrees of flexion).	☐	☐	☐
		Student applies stabilization to the opposite scapula.	☐	☐	☐
		Student instructs patient to: *(Hold your arm in this position and do not let me push it down).*	☐	☐	☐
		Student applies moderate resistance just proximal to the elbow.	☐	☐	☐
		Student grades the strength of the shoulder flexors and verbalizes it to instructor.	☐	☐	☐
		Student asks patient if they had any pain during that motion. If yes, student asks patient to rate their pain and documents the results.	☐	☐	☐

⚑ = Critical Safety Element/Professionalism. If a student is unable to complete a flagged step without cueing, they will need to return at another time to redo the check-off. All other steps can be cued.

	8	The student correctly measures **Shoulder Flexion MMT (gravity minimized):**			
		Student places patient in sidelying position with the upper extremity supported on a smooth surface and in neutral rotation, elbow flexed.	☐	☐	☐
		Student instructs patient to flex the shoulder through the range of motion. If no motion occurs at the joint, student palpates the muscle tendons to determine if there is a contraction.	☐	☐	☐
		Student grades the strength of the shoulder flexors and verbalizes it to instructor.	☐	☐	☐
		Student asks patient if they had any pain during that motion. If yes, student asks patient to rate their pain and documents the results.	☐	☐	☐
	9	The student correctly measures **Shoulder Extension MMT (against gravity):**			
		Student verbalizes the primary muscles they are assessing: *(Latissimus dorsi, teres major, posterior deltoid).*	☐	☐	☐
		Student places patient in a prone position with arms at side and palms facing the ceiling.	☐	☐	☐
		Student instructs patient to extend their shoulder through their full range of motion to ensure full active range of motion.	☐	☐	☐
		Student instructs patient to repeat that motion and then hold their arm in mid-range (20–30 degrees of extension).	☐	☐	☐
		Student applies stabilization to the ipsilateral border of the scapula staying off the spinous processes.	☐	☐	☐
		Student instructs patient to: *(Hold your arm in this position and do not let me push it down).*	☐	☐	☐
		Student applies moderate resistance just proximal to the elbow.	☐	☐	☐
		Student grades the strength of the shoulder extensors and verbalizes it to instructor.	☐	☐	☐
		Student asks patient if they had any pain during that motion. If yes, student asks patient to rate their pain and documents the results.	☐	☐	☐
	10	The student correctly measures **Shoulder Extension MMT (gravity minimized):**			
		Student places patient in sidelying position with the upper extremity supported on a smooth surface and in neutral rotation, elbow flexed.	☐	☐	☐
		Student instructs patient to extend the shoulder through the range of motion. If no motion occurs at the joint, student palpates the muscle tendons to determine if there is a contraction.	☐	☐	☐
		Student grades the strength of the shoulder extensor and verbalizes it to instructor.	☐	☐	☐
		Student asks patient if they had any pain during that motion. If yes, student asks patient to rate their pain and documents the results.	☐	☐	☐

☐ = Critical Safety Element/Professionalism. If a student is unable to complete a flagged step without cueing, they will need to return at another time to redo the check-off. All other steps can be cued.

	11	The student correctly measures **Shoulder Abduction MMT (against gravity)**:			
		Student verbalizes the primary muscle they are assessing: *(Middle deltoid).*	☐	☐	☐
		Student places patient in a seated position.	☐	☐	☐
		Student instructs patient to abduct their shoulder through their full range of motion to ensure full active range of motion.	☐	☐	☐
		Student instructs patient to repeat that motion and then hold their arm in mid-range, with palm down (90 degrees of abduction).	☐	☐	☐
		Student applies stabilization to the opposite shoulder.	☐	☐	☐
		Student instructs patient to: *(Hold your arm in this position and do not let me push it down).*	☐	☐	☐
		Student applies moderate resistance just proximal to the elbow.	☐	☐	☐
		Student grades the strength of the shoulder abductors and verbalizes it to instructor.	☐	☐	☐
		Student asks patient if they had any pain during that motion. If yes, student asks patient to rate their pain and documents the results.	☐	☐	☐
	12	The student correctly measures **Shoulder Abduction MMT (gravity minimized)**:			
		Student places patient in supine with limb resting on the table.	☐	☐	☐
		Student instructs patient to abduct the shoulder through the range of motion. If no motion occurs at the joint, student palpates the muscle tendons to determine if there is a contraction.	☐	☐	☐
		Student grades the strength of the shoulder abductors and verbalizes it to instructor.	☐	☐	☐
		Student asks patient if they had any pain during that motion. If yes, student asks patient to rate their pain and documents the results.	☐	☐	☐
	13	The student correctly measures **Shoulder Horizontal Abduction MMT (against gravity)**:			
		Student verbalizes the primary muscle they are assessing: *(Posterior deltoid).*	☐	☐	☐
		Student places patient in a prone position with the shoulder in 90 degrees of abduction with the forearm off the table and the elbow in flexion.	☐	☐	☐
		Student instructs patient to horizontally abduct their shoulder through their full range of motion to ensure full active range of motion.	☐	☐	☐
		Student instructs patient to repeat that motion and then hold their arm in mid-range (20 degrees of horizontal abduction).	☐	☐	☐
		Student applies stabilization to the ipsilateral scapula.	☐	☐	☐
		Student instructs patient to: *(Hold your arm in this position and do not let me push it down).*	☐	☐	☐
		Student applies moderate resistance just proximal to the elbow.	☐	☐	☐
		Student grades the strength of the shoulder horizontal abductors and verbalizes it to instructor.	☐	☐	☐
		Student asks patient if they had any pain during that motion. If yes, student asks patient to rate their pain and documents the results.	☐	☐	☐
	14	The student correctly measures **Shoulder Horizontal Abduction MMT (gravity minimized)**:			
		Student places patient in sitting with the arm supported on a table in 90 degrees of shoulder abduction with the elbow in flexion.	☐	☐	☐
		Student instructs patient to horizontally abduct the shoulder through the range of motion. If no motion occurs at the joint, student palpates the muscle tendons to determine if there is a contraction.	☐	☐	☐
		Student grades the strength of the shoulder horizontal abductors and verbalizes it to instructor.	☐	☐	☐
		Student asks patient if they had any pain during that motion. If yes, student asks patient to rate their pain and documents the results.	☐	☐	☐

☐ = Critical Safety Element/Professionalism. If a student is unable to complete a flagged step without cueing, they will need to return at another time to redo the check-off. All other steps can be cued.

	15	The student correctly measures **Shoulder Horizontal Adduction MMT (against gravity):**			
		Student verbalizes the primary muscle they are assessing: *(Pectoralis major).*	☐	☐	☐
		Student places patient in a supine position with the shoulder in 90 degrees of abduction, neutral rotation, and elbow flexed to 90 degrees.	☐	☐	☐
		Student instructs patient to horizontally adduct their shoulder through their full range of motion to ensure full active range of motion.	☐	☐	☐
		Student instructs patient to repeat that motion and then hold their arm in mid-range (45 degrees of horizontal adduction).	☐	☐	☐
		Student applies stabilization to the anterior aspect of the opposite shoulder.	☐	☐	☐
		Student instructs patient to: *(Hold your arm in this position and do not let me push it down).*	☐	☐	☐
		Student applies moderate resistance to the anterior medial aspect of the arm, just proximal to the elbow.	☐	☐	☐
		Student grades the strength of the shoulder horizontal adductors and verbalizes it to instructor.	☐	☐	☐
		Student asks patient if they had any pain during that motion. If yes, student asks patient to rate their pain and documents the results.	☐	☐	☐
	16	The student correctly measures **Shoulder Horizontal Adduction MMT (gravity minimized):**			
		Student places patient in sitting with the arm supported on a table in 90 degrees of shoulder abduction, neutral rotation, and the elbow flexed to 90 degrees.	☐	☐	☐
		Student instructs patient to horizontally adduct the shoulder through the range of motion. If no motion occurs at the joint, student palpates the muscle tendons to determine if there is a contraction.	☐	☐	☐
		Student grades the strength of the shoulder horizontal adductors and verbalizes it to instructor.	☐	☐	☐
		Student asks patient if they had any pain during that motion. If yes, student asks patient to rate their pain and documents the results.	☐	☐	☐
	17	The student correctly measures **Shoulder Internal Rotation MMT (against gravity):**			
		Student verbalizes the primary muscle they are assessing: *(Subscapularis).*	☐	☐	☐
		Student places patient in a prone position with the shoulder in 90 degrees of abduction and the elbow flexed over the edge of the table. Patient's head should be rotated to the tested side.	☐	☐	☐
		Student instructs patient to internally rotate their shoulder through their full range of motion to ensure full active range of motion.	☐	☐	☐
		Student instructs patient to repeat that motion and then hold their arm in mid-range (45 degrees of internal rotation).	☐	☐	☐
		Student applies stabilization to the humerus.	☐	☐	☐
		Student instructs patient to: *(Hold your arm in this position and do not let me push it down).*	☐	☐	☐
		Student applies moderate resistance to the flexor surface of the forearm, just proximal to the wrist.	☐	☐	☐
		Student grades the strength of the shoulder internal rotators and verbalizes it to instructor.	☐	☐	☐
		Student asks patient if they had any pain during that motion. If yes, student asks patient to rate their pain and documents the results.	☐	☐	☐

☐ = Critical Safety Element/Professionalism. If a student is unable to complete a flagged step without cueing, they will need to return at another time to redo the check-off. All other steps can be cued.

	18	The student correctly measures **Shoulder Internal Rotation MMT (gravity minimized):**			
		Student places patient in prone with the tested arm hanging freely over the edge of the table with the palm facing the table. The head should be rotated to the tested side.	☐	☐	☐
		Student instructs patient to internally rotate the shoulder through the range of motion. If no motion occurs at the joint, student palpates the muscle tendons to determine if there is a contraction.	☐	☐	☐
		Student grades the strength of the shoulder internal rotators and verbalizes it to instructor.	☐	☐	☐
		Student asks patient if they had any pain during that motion. If yes, student asks patient to rate their pain and documents the results.	☐	☐	☐
	19	The student correctly measures **Shoulder External Rotation MMT (against gravity):**			
		Student verbalizes the primary muscles they are assessing: *(Infraspinatus, teres minor).*	☐	☐	☐
		Student places patient in a prone position with the shoulder in 90 degrees of abduction and the elbow flexed over the edge of the table. Patient's head should be rotated to the tested side.	☐	☐	☐
		Student instructs patient to externally rotate their shoulder through their full range of motion to ensure full active range of motion.	☐	☐	☐
		Student instructs patient to repeat that motion and then hold their arm in mid-range (45 degrees of external rotation).	☐	☐	☐
		Student applies stabilization to the humerus.	☐	☐	☐
		Student instructs patient to: *(Hold your arm in this position and do not let me push it down).*	☐	☐	☐
		Student applies moderate resistance to the extensor surface of the forearm, just proximal to the wrist.	☐	☐	☐
		Student grades the strength of the shoulder external rotators and verbalizes it to instructor.	☐	☐	☐
		Student asks patient if they had any pain during that motion. If yes, student asks patient to rate their pain and documents the results.	☐	☐	☐
	20	The student correctly measures **Shoulder External Rotation MMT (gravity minimized):**			
		Student places patient in prone with the tested arm hanging freely over the edge of the table with the palm facing the table. The head should be rotated to the tested side.	☐	☐	☐
		Student instructs patient to externally rotate the shoulder through the range of motion. If no motion occurs at the joint, student palpates the muscle tendons to determine if there is a contraction.	☐	☐	☐
		Student grades the strength of the shoulder external rotators and verbalizes it to instructor.	☐	☐	☐
		Student asks patient if they had any pain during that motion. If yes, student asks patient to rate their pain and documents the results.	☐	☐	☐
Post-Skill	21	The student washes their hands post–skill performance:			
		Student removes all jewelry from their wrists and hands. Student turns the water to the preferred temperature and wets their hands. Student applies the soap to their hands and washes them with their hands pointed down. Student scrubs for 40–60 seconds and includes palm, between fingers, fingernails, and dorsum of hands. Student rinses hands with hands pointed down. Student dries their hands with a paper towel, uses a paper towel to turn off the water, and then disposes of the paper towel in the trash.	☐	☐	☐
	22	The student verbalizes that they will document their session in the note.	☐	☐	☐

⌐ = Critical Safety Element/Professionalism. If a student is unable to complete a flagged step without cueing, they will need to return at another time to redo the check-off. All other steps can be cued.

Other	23 ⚑	The student has optimal body mechanics during performance of the skill.	☐	☐	☐
	24 ⚑	The student uses appropriate therapeutic touch.	☐	☐	☐
	25	The student is able to complete the check-off in the time allotted.	☐	☐	☐
Communication	26	The student uses language the patient can understand.	☐	☐	☐
	27	The student listens actively to the patient during the session.	☐	☐	☐
	28	The student ensures the patient understands instructions by having the patient teach back or demonstrate.	☐	☐	☐
	29 ⚑	The student demonstrates confidence and provides the patient with clear instruction and cueing.	☐	☐	☐

Peer Name (Printed)		**Peer Signature**		**Date of Peer Review**	
Instructor Name (Printed and Signature)	By signing this skills checklist, I am declaring this student competent in the skill described above.			**Date of Instructor Review**	
NOTES					

⚑ = Critical Safety Element/Professionalism. If a student is unable to complete a flagged step without cueing, they will need to return at another time to redo the check-off. All other steps can be cued.

Student Name: _____

Skill		Manual Muscle Testing: Elbow/Forearm			
Source		Van Ost L, Morogiello J. *Cram Session in Goniometry and Manual Muscle Testing:* *A Handbook for Students & Clinicians.* 2nd ed. SLACK Incorporated; 2023.	**Check When Completed**		
			Self	Peer	Instructor
Student Introduction and Consent	1 ⚑	The student introduces themself to the patient. Must include that they are a **student** PTA and list the school's name.	☐	☐	☐
	2 ⚑	The student verifies the patient's identity. Must use at least 2 patient identifiers (name, date of birth).	☐	☐	☐
	3 ⚑	The student gains consent: • Speaks with the patient about their status (acquires relevant information) • Educates the patient on intended data collection/intervention and goals for the session • Gains permission to perform said data collection/intervention	☐	☐	☐
Student, Patient, and Supply Preparation	4 ⚑	The student gathers supplies and prepares treatment area (cleans equipment, checks for safety hazards, ensures all equipment is functional and appropriate).	☐	☐	☐
	5	The student washes their hands:			
		Student removes all jewelry from their wrists and hands. Student turns the water to the preferred temperature and wets their hands. Student applies the soap to their hands and washes them with their hands pointed down. Student scrubs for 40–60 seconds and includes palm, between fingers, fingernails, and dorsum of hands. Student rinses hands with hands pointed down. Student dries their hands with a paper towel, uses a paper towel to turn off the water, and then disposes of the paper towel in the trash.	☐	☐	☐
	6	The student places the patient in the correct position for support, comfort, and access to body area necessary for data collection/intervention.	☐	☐	☐
Skill Performance	7	The student correctly measures **Elbow Flexion MMT (against gravity)**:			
		Student verbalizes the primary muscles they are assessing: *(Biceps brachii, brachialis, brachioradialis).*	☐	☐	☐
		Student places patient in a seated position.	☐	☐	☐
		Student instructs patient to flex their elbow with their forearm supinated through their full range of motion to ensure full active range of motion.	☐	☐	☐
		Student instructs patient to repeat that motion and then hold their arm in mid-range (90 degrees of flexion).	☐	☐	☐
		Student stabilizes the upper arm against the trunk.	☐	☐	☐
		Student instructs patient to: *(Hold your arm in this position and do not let me push it down).*	☐	☐	☐
		Student applies moderate resistance to the anterior forearm just proximal to the elbow. Student repeats the test with forearm pronated (brachialis) and with forearm in neutral (brachioradialis).	☐	☐	☐
		Student grades the strength of the elbow flexors and verbalizes it to instructor.	☐	☐	☐
		Student asks patient if they had any pain during that motion. If yes, student asks patient to rate their pain and documents the results.	☐	☐	☐

⚑ = Critical Safety Element/Professionalism. If a student is unable to complete a flagged step without cueing, they will need to return at another time to redo the check-off. All other steps can be cued.

	8	The student correctly measures **Elbow Flexion MMT (gravity minimized):**			
		Student places patient in sitting with the upper extremity resting on a smooth surface. The shoulder is in 90 degrees of abduction with the elbow in maximal extension and forearm in neutral.	☐	☐	☐
		Student instructs patient to flex the elbow through the range of motion. If no motion occurs at the joint, student palpates the muscle tendons to determine if there is a contraction.	☐	☐	☐
		Student grades the strength of the elbow flexors and verbalizes it to instructor.	☐	☐	☐
		Student asks patient if they had any pain during that motion. If yes, student asks patient to rate their pain and documents the results.	☐	☐	☐
	9	The student correctly measures **Elbow Extension MMT (against gravity):**			
		Student verbalizes the primary muscles they are assessing: *(Triceps brachii, anconeus).*	☐	☐	☐
		Student places patient in a supine position with the shoulder flexed to 90 degrees and the elbow in maximal flexion.	☐	☐	☐
		Student instructs patient to extend their elbow through their full range of motion to ensure full active range of motion.	☐	☐	☐
		Student instructs patient to repeat that motion and then hold their arm in mid-range (90 degrees of flexion).	☐	☐	☐
		Student applies stabilization to the posterior aspect of the upper arm.	☐	☐	☐
		Student instructs patient to: *(Hold your arm in this position and do not let me push it down).*	☐	☐	☐
		Student applies moderate resistance just proximal to the wrist.	☐	☐	☐
		Student grades the strength of the elbow extensors and verbalizes it to instructor.	☐	☐	☐
		Student asks patient if they had any pain during that motion. If yes, student asks patient to rate their pain and documents the results.	☐	☐	☐
	10	The student correctly measures **Elbow Extension MMT (gravity minimized):**			
		Student places patient in sitting with the upper extremity resting on a smooth surface. The shoulder should be in 90 degrees of abduction and internally rotated with the elbow in maximal flexion and forearm in neutral or pronated.	☐	☐	☐
		Student instructs patient to extend the elbow through the range of motion. If no motion occurs at the joint, student palpates the muscle tendons to determine if there is a contraction.	☐	☐	☐
		Student grades the strength of the elbow extensors and verbalizes it to instructor.	☐	☐	☐
		Student asks patient if they had any pain during that motion. If yes, student asks patient to rate their pain and documents the results.	☐	☐	☐

☐ = Critical Safety Element/Professionalism. If a student is unable to complete a flagged step without cueing, they will need to return at another time to redo the check-off. All other steps can be cued.

	11	The student correctly measures **Forearm Supination MMT (against gravity)**:			
		Student verbalizes the primary muscles they are assessing: *(Supinator).*	☐	☐	☐
		Student places patient in a seated position with elbow flexed and forearm in pronation.	☐	☐	☐
		Student instructs patient to supinate their forearm through their full range of motion to ensure full active range of motion.	☐	☐	☐
		Student instructs patient to repeat that motion and then hold their arm in mid-range, with palm down (45 degrees of supination).	☐	☐	☐
		Student stabilizes the upper arm against the trunk.	☐	☐	☐
		Student instructs patient to: *(Hold your arm in this position and do not let me move it).*	☐	☐	☐
		Student applies moderate resistance to the wrist just proximal to the joint line into pronation.	☐	☐	☐
		Student grades the strength of the forearm supinators and verbalizes it to instructor.	☐	☐	☐
		Student asks patient if they had any pain during that motion. If yes, student asks patient to rate their pain and documents the results.	☐	☐	☐
	12	The student correctly measures **Forearm Supination MMT (gravity minimized)**:			
		Student places patient in sitting with the shoulder approximately 45 degrees of flexion, the elbow flexed, and the forearm in neutral. The student supports the arm at the elbow.	☐	☐	☐
		Student instructs patient to supinate the forearm through the range of motion. If no motion occurs at the joint, student palpates the muscle tendons to determine if there is a contraction.	☐	☐	☐
		Student grades the strength of the forearm supinators and verbalizes it to instructor.	☐	☐	☐
		Student asks patient if they had any pain during that motion. If yes, student asks patient to rate their pain and documents the results.	☐	☐	☐
	13	The student correctly measures **Forearm Pronation MMT (against gravity)**:			
		Student verbalizes the primary muscles they are assessing: *(Pronator teres, pronator quadratus).*	☐	☐	☐
		Student places patient in a seated position with elbow flexed and forearm in supination.	☐	☐	☐
		Student instructs patient to pronate their forearm through their full range of motion to ensure full active range of motion.	☐	☐	☐
		Student instructs patient to repeat that motion and then hold their arm in mid-range, with palm down (45 degrees of pronation).	☐	☐	☐
		Student stabilizes the upper arm against the trunk.	☐	☐	☐
		Student instructs patient to: *(Hold your arm in this position and do not let me move it).*	☐	☐	☐
		Student applies moderate resistance to the wrist just proximal to the joint line into supination.	☐	☐	☐
		Student grades the strength of the forearm pronators and verbalizes it to instructor.	☐	☐	☐
		Student asks patient if they had any pain during that motion. If yes, student asks patient to rate their pain and documents the results.	☐	☐	☐

☐ = Critical Safety Element/Professionalism. If a student is unable to complete a flagged step without cueing, they will need to return at another time to redo the check-off. All other steps can be cued.

	14	The student correctly measures **Forearm Pronation MMT (gravity minimized):**			
		Student places patient in sitting with the shoulder approximately 45 degrees of flexion, the elbow flexed, and the forearm in neutral. Student supports the arm at the elbow.	☐	☐	☐
		Student instructs patient to pronate the forearm through the range of motion. If no motion occurs at the joint, student palpates the muscle tendons to determine if there is a contraction.	☐	☐	☐
		Student grades the strength of the forearm pronators and verbalizes it to instructor.	☐	☐	☐
		Student asks patient if they had any pain during that motion. If yes, student asks patient to rate their pain and documents the results.	☐	☐	☐
Post-Skill	15	The student washes their hands post–skill performance:			
		Student removes all jewelry from their wrists and hands. Student turns the water to the preferred temperature and wets their hands. Student applies the soap to their hands and washes them with their hands pointed down. Student scrubs for 40–60 seconds and includes palm, between fingers, fingernails, and dorsum of hands. Student rinses hands with hands pointed down. Student dries their hands with a paper towel, uses a paper towel to turn off the water, and then disposes of the paper towel in the trash.	☐	☐	☐
	16	The student verbalizes that they will document their session in the note.	☐	☐	☐
Other	17 ⌐	The student has optimal body mechanics during performance of the skill.	☐	☐	☐
	18 ⌐	The student uses appropriate therapeutic touch.	☐	☐	☐
	19	The student is able to complete the check-off in the time allotted.	☐	☐	☐
Communication	20	The student uses language the patient can understand.	☐	☐	☐
	21	The student listens actively to the patient during the session.	☐	☐	☐
	22	The student ensures the patient understands instructions by having the patient teach back or demonstrate.	☐	☐	☐
	23 ⌐	The student demonstrates confidence and provides the patient with clear instruction and cueing.	☐	☐	☐

Peer Name (Printed)		**Peer Signature**		**Date of Peer Review**	
Instructor Name (Printed and Signature)	By signing this skills checklist, I am declaring this student competent in the skill described above.			**Date of Instructor Review**	
NOTES					

⌐ = Critical Safety Element/Professionalism. If a student is unable to complete a flagged step without cueing, they will need to return at another time to redo the check-off. All other steps can be cued.

Student Name: _____

Skill		Manual Muscle Testing: Wrist			
Source		Van Ost L, Morogiello J. *Cram Session in Goniometry and Manual Muscle Testing: A Handbook for Students & Clinicians*. 2nd ed. SLACK Incorporated; 2023.	Check When Completed		
			Self	Peer	Instructor
Student Introduction and Consent	1 ⚑	The student introduces themself to the patient. Must include that they are a **student** PTA and list the school's name.	☐	☐	☐
	2 ⚑	The student verifies the patient's identity. Must use at least 2 patient identifiers (name, date of birth).	☐	☐	☐
	3 ⚑	The student gains consent: • Speaks with the patient about their status (acquires relevant information) • Educates the patient on intended data collection/intervention and goals for the session • Gains permission to perform said data collection/intervention	☐	☐	☐
Student, Patient, and Supply Preparation	4 ⚑	The student gathers supplies and prepares treatment area (cleans equipment, checks for safety hazards, ensures all equipment is functional and appropriate).	☐	☐	☐
	5	The student washes their hands:			
		Student removes all jewelry from their wrists and hands. Student turns the water to the preferred temperature and wets their hands. Student applies the soap to their hands and washes them with their hands pointed down. Student scrubs for 40–60 seconds and includes palm, between fingers, fingernails, and dorsum of hands. Student rinses hands with hands pointed down. Student dries their hands with a paper towel, uses a paper towel to turn off the water, and then disposes of the paper towel in the trash.	☐	☐	☐
	6	The student places the patient in the correct position for support, comfort, and access to body area necessary for data collection/intervention.	☐	☐	☐
Skill Performance	7	The student correctly measures **Wrist Flexion MMT (against gravity)**:			
		Student verbalizes the primary muscles they are assessing: *(Flexor carpi radialis, flexor carpi ulnaris)*.	☐	☐	☐
		Student places patient seated with the forearm supinated and the dorsal surface resting on a tabletop. The wrist should be neutral, with the fingers relaxed.	☐	☐	☐
		Student instructs patient to flex their wrist through their full range of motion to ensure full active range of motion.	☐	☐	☐
		Student instructs patient to repeat that motion and then hold their arm in mid-range (45 degrees of flexion).	☐	☐	☐
		Student stabilizes the forearm against the tabletop.	☐	☐	☐
		Student instructs patient to: *(Hold your arm in this position and do not let me move it)*.	☐	☐	☐
		Student applies moderate resistance to the palm into wrist extension.	☐	☐	☐
		Student grades the strength of the wrist flexors and verbalizes it to instructor.	☐	☐	☐
		Student asks patient if they had any pain during that motion. If yes, student asks patient to rate their pain and documents the results.	☐	☐	☐

⚑ = Critical Safety Element/Professionalism. If a student is unable to complete a flagged step without cueing, they will need to return at another time to redo the check-off. All other steps can be cued.

	8	The student correctly measures **Wrist Flexion MMT (gravity minimized)**:			
		Student places patient in sitting with the forearm in neutral and the ulnar border of the hand resting on a tabletop with the wrist in neutral. The fingers should be relaxed.	☐	☐	☐
		Student instructs patient to flex the wrist through the range of motion. If no motion occurs at the joint, student palpates the muscle tendons to determine if there is a contraction.	☐	☐	☐
		Student grades the strength of the wrist flexors and verbalizes it to instructor.	☐	☐	☐
		Student asks patient if they had any pain during that motion. If yes, student asks patient to rate their pain and documents the results.	☐	☐	☐
	9	The student correctly measures **Wrist Extension MMT (against gravity)**:			
		Student verbalizes the primary muscles they are assessing: *(Extensor carpi radialis longus, extensor carpi radialis brevis, extensor carpi ulnaris).*	☐	☐	☐
		Student places patient in a seated position with the forearm pronated. The wrist should be neutral, with the fingers relaxed.	☐	☐	☐
		Student instructs patient to extend their wrist through their full range of motion to ensure full active range of motion.	☐	☐	☐
		Student instructs patient to repeat that motion and then hold their arm in mid-range (35 degrees of extension).	☐	☐	☐
		Student stabilizes the forearm against the tabletop.	☐	☐	☐
		Student instructs patient to: *(Hold your arm in this position and do not let me move it).*	☐	☐	☐
		Student applies moderate resistance to the dorsum of the hand into wrist flexion.	☐	☐	☐
		Student grades the strength of the wrist extensors and verbalizes it to instructor.	☐	☐	☐
		Student asks patient if they had any pain during that motion. If yes, student asks patient to rate their pain and documents the results.	☐	☐	☐
	10	The student correctly measures **Wrist Extension MMT (gravity minimized)**:			
		Student places patient in sitting with the forearm in neutral and the ulnar border of the hand resting on a tabletop with the wrist in neutral. The fingers should be relaxed.	☐	☐	☐
		Student instructs patient to extend the wrist through the range of motion. If no motion occurs at the joint, student palpates the muscle tendons to determine if there is a contraction.	☐	☐	☐
		Student grades the strength of the wrist extensors and verbalizes it to instructor.	☐	☐	☐
		Student asks patient if they had any pain during that motion. If yes, student asks patient to rate their pain and documents the results.	☐	☐	☐
Post-Skill	11	The student washes their hands post–skill performance:			
		Student removes all jewelry from their wrists and hands. Student turns the water to the preferred temperature and wets their hands. Student applies the soap to their hands and washes them with their hands pointed down. Student scrubs for 40–60 seconds and includes palm, between fingers, fingernails, and dorsum of hands. Student rinses hands with hands pointed down. Student dries their hands with a paper towel, uses a paper towel to turn off the water, and then disposes of the paper towel in the trash.	☐	☐	☐
	12	The student verbalizes that they will document their session in the note.	☐	☐	☐
Other	13 ⚑	The student has optimal body mechanics during performance of the skill.	☐	☐	☐
	14 ⚑	The student uses appropriate therapeutic touch.	☐	☐	☐
	15	The student is able to complete the check-off in the time allotted.	☐	☐	☐

⚑ = Critical Safety Element/Professionalism. If a student is unable to complete a flagged step without cueing, they will need to return at another time to redo the check-off. All other steps can be cued.

Communication	16	The student uses language the patient can understand.		☐	☐	☐
	17	The student listens actively to the patient during the session.		☐	☐	☐
	18	The student ensures the patient understands instructions by having the patient teach back or demonstrate.		☐	☐	☐
	19 ⚑	The student demonstrates confidence and provides the patient with clear instruction and cueing.		☐	☐	☐

Peer Name (Printed)		Peer Signature		Date of Peer Review	
Instructor Name (Printed and Signature)	By signing this skills checklist, I am declaring this student competent in the skill described above.			Date of Instructor Review	
NOTES					

⚑ = Critical Safety Element/Professionalism. If a student is unable to complete a flagged step without cueing, they will need to return at another time to redo the check-off. All other steps can be cued.

Student Name: _____

Skill		Manual Muscle Testing: Trunk			
Source		Van Ost L, Morogiello J. *Cram Session in Goniometry and Manual Muscle Testing: A Handbook for Students & Clinicians*. 2nd ed. SLACK Incorporated; 2023.	**Check When Completed**		
			Self	Peer	Instructor
Student Introduction and Consent	1 ⚑	The student introduces themself to the patient. Must include that they are a **student** PTA and list the school's name.	☐	☐	☐
	2 ⚑	The student verifies the patient's identity. Must use at least 2 patient identifiers (name, date of birth).	☐	☐	☐
	3 ⚑	The student gains consent: <ul><li>Speaks with the patient about their status (acquires relevant information)</li><li>Educates the patient on intended data collection/intervention and goals for the session</li><li>Gains permission to perform said data collection/intervention</li></ul>	☐	☐	☐
Student, Patient, and Supply Preparation	4 ⚑	The student gathers supplies and prepares treatment area (cleans equipment, checks for safety hazards, ensures all equipment is functional and appropriate).	☐	☐	☐
	5	The student washes their hands:			
		Student removes all jewelry from their wrists and hands. Student turns the water to the preferred temperature and wets their hands. Student applies the soap to their hands and washes them with their hands pointed down. Student scrubs for 40–60 seconds and includes palm, between fingers, fingernails, and dorsum of hands. Student rinses hands with hands pointed down. Student dries their hands with a paper towel, uses a paper towel to turn off the water, and then disposes of the paper towel in the trash.	☐	☐	☐
	6	The student places the patient in the correct position for support, comfort, and access to body area necessary for data collection/intervention.	☐	☐	☐
Skill Performance	7	The student correctly measures **Trunk Flexion MMT**:			
		Student verbalizes the primary muscles they are assessing: *(Rectus abdominis, external oblique, internal oblique)*.	☐	☐	☐
		Student places patient in a supine position with both lower extremities in extension.	☐	☐	☐
		Student explains to patient they will be asking them to perform different movements to determine their general trunk flexion strength.	☐	☐	☐
		Student instructs patient to place their hands behind their head.	☐	☐	☐
		Student instructs patient to curl their head, shoulders, and torso up until their shoulder blades are off the table.	☐	☐	☐
		Student provides light stabilization on the thigh nearest to them.	☐	☐	☐
		If patient can clear the scapula completely, student will grade them a 5/5, document their results, and continue with their treatment session. If patient is unable to clear the scapula completely, student will assess patient for 4/5 strength.	☐	☐	☐
		Student instructs patient to cross their hands over their chest.	☐	☐	☐
		Student instructs patient to curl their head, shoulders, and torso up until their shoulder blades are off the table.	☐	☐	☐

⚑ = Critical Safety Element/Professionalism. If a student is unable to complete a flagged step without cueing, they will need to return at another time to redo the check-off. All other steps can be cued.

		Student provides light stabilization on the thigh nearest to them.	☐	☐	☐
		If patient can clear the scapula completely, student will grade them a 4/5, document their results, and continue with their treatment session. If patient is unable to clear the scapula completely, student will assess patient for 3/5 strength.	☐	☐	☐
		Student instructs patient to extend their arms over the trunk.	☐	☐	☐
		Student instructs patient to curl their head, shoulders, and torso up until their shoulder blades are off the table.	☐	☐	☐
		Student provides light stabilization on the thigh nearest to them.	☐	☐	☐
		If patient can clear the scapula completely, student will grade them a 3/5, document their results, and continue with their treatment session. If patient is unable to clear the scapula completely, student will assess patient for 2/5 strength.	☐	☐	☐
		Student instructs patient to place their arms by their sides on the mat table.	☐	☐	☐
		Student instructs patient to curl their head, shoulders, and torso up until their shoulder blades are off the table, sliding their hands along the mat.	☐	☐	☐
		Student provides light stabilization on the thigh nearest to them.	☐	☐	☐
		If patient can lift their head and neck off the mat table but are unable to clear the scapula completely, student will grade them a 2/5, document their results, and continue with their treatment session. If patient is unable to lift their head and neck off the mat table, student will assess patient for 1/5 strength.	☐	☐	☐
		Student instructs patient to curl their head, shoulders, and torso up until their shoulder blades are off the table, sliding their hands along the mat.	☐	☐	☐
		Student provides light stabilization on the thigh nearest to them.	☐	☐	☐
		If patient is unable able to lift their head and neck off the mat table but student can feel muscle activity to the rectus abdominis, student will grade them a 1/5, document their results, and continue with their treatment session. If patient is unable to lift their head and neck off the mat table and there is no muscle activation by the rectus abdominis, student will grade them a 0/5, document their results, and continue with their treatment session.	☐	☐	☐
		Student asks patient if they had any pain during that motion. If yes, student asks patient to rate their pain and documents the results.	☐	☐	☐
	8	The student correctly measures **Trunk Rotation MMT**:			
		Student verbalizes the primary muscles they are assessing: *(External oblique, internal oblique).*	☐	☐	☐
		Student places patient in a supine position with both lower extremities in extension.	☐	☐	☐
		Student explains to patient they will be asking them to perform different movements to determine their general trunk rotation strength.	☐	☐	☐
		Student instructs patient to place their hands behind their head.	☐	☐	☐
		Student instructs patient to lift their head and shoulders off the table and turn their left elbow toward their right knee.	☐	☐	☐
		Student provides light stabilization on the pelvis.	☐	☐	☐

☐ = Critical Safety Element/Professionalism. If a student is unable to complete a flagged step without cueing, they will need to return at another time to redo the check-off. All other steps can be cued.

		If patient can clear the scapula completely, student will grade them a 5/5, document their results, and continue with their treatment session. If patient is unable to clear the scapula completely, student will assess patient for 4/5 strength.	☐	☐	☐
		Student instructs patient to cross their hands over their chest.	☐	☐	☐
		Student instructs patient to lift their head and shoulders off the table and turn their left elbow toward their right knee.	☐	☐	☐
		Student provides light stabilization on the pelvis.	☐	☐	☐
		If patient can clear the scapula completely, student will grade them a 4/5, document their results, and continue with their treatment session. If patient is unable to clear the scapula completely, student will assess patient for 3/5 strength.	☐	☐	☐
		Student instructs patient to extend their arms.	☐	☐	☐
		Student instructs patient to lift their head and shoulders off the table and reach toward their right knee.	☐	☐	☐
		Student provides light stabilization on the pelvis.	☐	☐	☐
		If patient can clear the scapula completely, student will grade them a 3/5, document their results, and continue with their treatment session. If patient is unable to clear the scapula completely, student will assess patient for 2/5 strength.	☐	☐	☐
		Student instructs patient to place their arms by their sides on the mat table.	☐	☐	☐
		Student instructs patient to lift their head and shoulders off the table and turn their left shoulder toward their right knee.	☐	☐	☐
		Student provides light stabilization on the pelvis.	☐	☐	☐
		If patient can lift their head and neck off the mat table but are unable to clear the scapula completely, student will grade them a 2/5, document their results, and continue with their treatment session. If patient is unable to lift their head and neck off the mat table, student will assess patient for 1/5 strength.	☐	☐	☐
		Student instructs patient to lift their head and shoulders off the table and turn their left shoulder toward their right knee.	☐	☐	☐
		Student provides light stabilization on the pelvis.	☐	☐	☐
		If patient is unable able to lift their head and neck off the mat table but student can feel muscle activity to the rectus abdominis, student will grade them a 1/5, document their results, and continue with their treatment session. If patient is unable to lift their head and neck off the mat table and there is no muscle activation by the rectus abdominis, student will grade them a 0/5, document their results, and continue with their treatment session.	☐	☐	☐
		Student asks patient if they had any pain during that motion. If yes, student asks patient to rate their pain and documents the results.	☐	☐	☐

⌐ = Critical Safety Element/Professionalism. If a student is unable to complete a flagged step without cueing, they will need to return at another time to redo the check-off. All other steps can be cued.

	9	The student correctly measures **Trunk Extension MMT**:			
		Student verbalizes the primary muscles they are assessing: *(Iliocostalis thoracis, longissimus thoracis, semispinalis thoracis, multifidi, rotatores thoracis and lumborum, interspinales thoracis and lumborum, intertransversarii thoracis and lumborum, quadratus lumborum).*	☐	☐	☐
		Student places patient in a prone position with both lower extremities in extension.	☐	☐	☐
		Student explains to patient that they will be asking them to perform different movements to determine their general trunk extension strength.	☐	☐	☐
		Student instructs patient to place their hands behind their head.	☐	☐	☐
		Student instructs patient to lift their head and chest up toward the ceiling as high as possible and hold it.	☐	☐	☐
		Student provides moderate stabilization to the pelvis and hips.	☐	☐	☐
		If patient can clear the sternum completely, student will grade them a 5/5, document their results, and continue with their treatment session. If patient is unable to clear the sternum completely, student will assess patient for 4/5 strength.	☐	☐	☐
		Student instructs patient to place their hands behind their back on the lumbar spine.	☐	☐	☐
		Student instructs patient to lift their head and chest up toward the ceiling as high as possible and hold it.	☐	☐	☐
		Student provides moderate stabilization to the pelvis and hips.	☐	☐	☐
		If patient can clear the sternum completely, student will grade them a 4/5, document their results, and continue with their treatment session. If patient is unable to clear the sternum completely, student will assess them for 3/5 strength.	☐	☐	☐
		Student instructs patient to place their arms by their sides on the mat table, palms up.	☐	☐	☐
		Student instructs patient to lift their head and chest up toward the ceiling as high as possible and hold it.	☐	☐	☐
		Student provides moderate stabilization to the pelvis and hips.	☐	☐	☐
		If patient can clear the sternum completely, student will grade them a 3/5, document their results, and continue with their treatment session. If patient is unable to clear the sternum completely, student will assess them for 2/5 strength.	☐	☐	☐
		Student instructs patient to place their arms by their sides on the mat table, palms up.	☐	☐	☐
		Student instructs the patient to lift their head and chest up toward the ceiling as high as possible and hold it.	☐	☐	☐
		Student provides moderate stabilization to the pelvis and hips.	☐	☐	☐
		If patient can lift their head and shoulders off the mat table, but unable to clear the sternum completely, student will grade them a 2/5, document their results, and continue with their treatment session. If patient is unable to lift their head and shoulders off the mat table, student will assess them for 1/5 strength.	☐	☐	☐
		Student instructs patient to place their arms by their sides on the mat table, palms up.	☐	☐	☐
		Student instructs patient to lift their head and chest up toward the ceiling as high as possible and hold it.	☐	☐	☐

◻ = Critical Safety Element/Professionalism. If a student is unable to complete a flagged step without cueing, they will need to return at another time to redo the check-off. All other steps can be cued.

		Student provides moderate stabilization to the pelvis and hips.	☐	☐	☐
		If patient is unable to lift their head and shoulders off the mat table but student can palpate muscle activity at the erector spinae, student will grade them a 1/5, document their results, and continue with their treatment session. If patient is unable to lift their head and shoulders off the mat table and student does not feel any muscle activation at the erector spinae, student will grade them a 0/5, document their results, and continue with their treatment session.	☐	☐	☐
		Student asks patient if they had any pain during that motion. If yes, student asks patient to rate their pain and documents the results.	☐	☐	☐
Post-Skill	10	The student washes their hands post–skill performance:			
		Student removes all jewelry from their wrists and hands. Student turns the water to the preferred temperature and wets their hands. Student applies the soap to their hands and washes them with their hands pointed down. Student scrubs for 40–60 seconds and includes palm, between fingers, fingernails, and dorsum of hands. Student rinses hands with hands pointed down. Student dries their hands with a paper towel, uses a paper towel to turn off the water, and then disposes of the paper towel in the trash.	☐	☐	☐
	11	The student verbalizes that they will document their session in the note.	☐	☐	☐
Other	12 ⚑	The student has optimal body mechanics during performance of the skill.	☐	☐	☐
	13 ⚑	The student uses appropriate therapeutic touch.	☐	☐	☐
	14	The student is able to complete the check-off in the time allotted.	☐	☐	☐
Communication	15	The student uses language the patient can understand.	☐	☐	☐
	16	The student listens actively to the patient during the session.	☐	☐	☐
	17	The student ensures the patient understands instructions by having the patient teach back or demonstrate.	☐	☐	☐
	18 ⚑	The student demonstrates confidence and provides the patient with clear instruction and cueing.	☐	☐	☐

Peer Name (Printed)		Peer Signature		Date of Peer Review	
Instructor Name (Printed and Signature)	By signing this skills checklist, I am declaring this student competent in the skill described above.			Date of Instructor Review	
NOTES					

⚑ = Critical Safety Element/Professionalism. If a student is unable to complete a flagged step without cueing, they will need to return at another time to redo the check-off. All other steps can be cued.

Student Name: _____

Skill		Manual Muscle Testing: Hip			
Source		Van Ost L, Morogiello J. *Cram Session in Goniometry and Manual Muscle Testing: A Handbook for Students & Clinicians*. 2nd ed. SLACK Incorporated; 2023.	Check When Completed		
			Self	Peer	Instructor
Student Introduction and Consent	1 ⚑	The student introduces themself to the patient. Must include that they are a **student** PTA and list the school's name.	☐	☐	☐
	2 ⚑	The student verifies the patient's identity. Must use at least 2 patient identifiers (name, date of birth).	☐	☐	☐
	3 ⚑	The student gains consent: • Speaks with the patient about their status (acquires relevant information) • Educates the patient on intended data collection/intervention and goals for the session • Gains permission to perform said data collection/intervention	☐	☐	☐
Student, Patient, and Supply Preparation	4 ⚑	The student gathers supplies and prepares treatment area (cleans equipment, checks for safety hazards, ensures all equipment is functional and appropriate).	☐	☐	☐
	5	The student washes their hands:			
		Student removes all jewelry from their wrists and hands. Student turns the water to the preferred temperature and wets their hands. Student applies the soap to their hands and washes them with their hands pointed down. Student scrubs for 40–60 seconds and includes palm, between fingers, fingernails, and dorsum of hands. Student rinses hands with hands pointed down. Student dries their hands with a paper towel, uses a paper towel to turn off the water, and then disposes of the paper towel in the trash.	☐	☐	☐
	6	The student places the patient in the correct position for support, comfort, and access to body area necessary for data collection/intervention.	☐	☐	☐
Skill Performance	7	The student correctly measures **Hip Flexion MMT (against gravity)**:			
		Student verbalizes the primary muscles they are assessing: *(Psoas major, iliacus).*	☐	☐	☐
		Student places patient in a seated position with legs off the bed's edge, hands on the table for stability.	☐	☐	☐
		Student instructs patient to flex their hip through their full range of motion to ensure full active range of motion.	☐	☐	☐
		Student instructs patient to repeat that motion and then hold their hip in mid-range (100 degrees of flexion).	☐	☐	☐
		Student applies stabilization to the opposite side of the pelvis.	☐	☐	☐
		Student instructs patient to: *(Hold your leg in this position and do not let me push it down).*	☐	☐	☐
		Student applies moderate resistance over the distal thigh just proximal to the knee joint.	☐	☐	☐
		Student grades the strength of the hip flexors and verbalizes it to instructor.	☐	☐	☐
		Student asks patient if they had any pain during that motion. If yes, student asks patient to rate their pain and documents the results.	☐	☐	☐

⚑ = Critical Safety Element/Professionalism. If a student is unable to complete a flagged step without cueing, they will need to return at another time to redo the check-off. All other steps can be cued.

	8	The student correctly measures **Hip Flexion MMT (gravity minimized)**:			
		Student places patient in sidelying position with the tested limb resting on a powder board with the hip in neutral and the knee flexed to 90 degrees or with the clinician supporting the tested limb.	☐	☐	☐
		Student instructs patient to flex the hip through the range of motion. If no motion occurs at the joint, student palpates the muscle tendons to determine if there is a contraction.	☐	☐	☐
		Student grades the strength of the hip flexors and verbalizes it to instructor.	☐	☐	☐
		Student asks patient if they had any pain during that motion. If yes, student asks patient to rate their pain and documents the results.	☐	☐	☐
	9	The student correctly measures **Hip Extension MMT (against gravity)**:			
		Student verbalizes the primary muscles they are assessing: *(Gluteus maximus, semitendinosus, semimembranosus, biceps femoris)*.	☐	☐	☐
		Student places patient in a prone position with arms by the sides and the lower extremities extended.	☐	☐	☐
		Student instructs patient to extend their hip through their full range of motion to ensure full active range of motion.	☐	☐	☐
		Student instructs patient to repeat that motion and then hold their leg in mid-range (10 degrees of extension).	☐	☐	☐
		Student applies stabilization to the ipsilateral pelvis against the table.	☐	☐	☐
		Student instructs patient to: *(Hold your leg in this position and do not let me push it down)*.	☐	☐	☐
		Student applies moderate resistance to the posterior thigh just proximal to the knee.	☐	☐	☐
		Student grades the strength of the hip extensors and verbalizes it to instructor.	☐	☐	☐
		Student asks patient if they had any pain during that motion. If yes, student asks patient to rate their pain and documents the results.	☐	☐	☐
	10	The student correctly measures **Hip Extension MMT (gravity minimized)**:			
		Student places patient in sidelying position with the tested limb on top supported on a powder board or supported by the clinician. The knee is positioned loosely in extension and the bottom hip and knee are flexed for stability.	☐	☐	☐
		Student instructs patient to extend the hip through the range of motion. If no motion occurs at the joint, student palpates the muscle tendons to determine if there is a contraction.	☐	☐	☐
		Student grades the strength of the hip extensors and verbalizes it to instructor.	☐	☐	☐
		Student asks patient if they had any pain during that motion. If yes, student asks patient to rate their pain and documents the results.	☐	☐	☐
	11	The student correctly measures **Hip Abduction MMT (against gravity)**:			
		Student verbalizes the primary muscles they are assessing: *(Gluteus medius, gluteus minimus)*.	☐	☐	☐
		Student places patient in a sidelying position with the bottom hip and knee flexed for stability, the tested limb lies on top with the hip and knee extended in neutral.	☐	☐	☐
		Student instructs patient to abduct their hip through their full range of motion to ensure full active range of motion.	☐	☐	☐
		Student instructs patient to repeat that motion and then hold their leg in mid-range (20–30 degrees of abduction).	☐	☐	☐
		Student applies stabilization to the ipsilateral pelvis.	☐	☐	☐
		Student instructs patient to: *(Hold your leg in this position and do not let me push it down)*.	☐	☐	☐
		Student applies moderate resistance on the lateral aspect of the thigh just proximal to the knee joint.	☐	☐	☐
		Student grades the strength of the hip abductors and verbalizes it to instructor.	☐	☐	☐
		Student asks patient if they had any pain during that motion. If yes, student asks patient to rate their pain and documents the results.	☐	☐	☐

☐ = Critical Safety Element/Professionalism. If a student is unable to complete a flagged step without cueing, they will need to return at another time to redo the check-off. All other steps can be cued.

	12	The student correctly measures **Hip Abduction MMT (gravity minimized)**:			
		Student places patient supine with the tested limb in extension resting on a smooth surface supported by student.	☐	☐	☐
		Student instructs patient to abduct the hip through the range of motion. If no motion occurs at the joint, student palpates the muscle tendons to determine if there is a contraction.	☐	☐	☐
		Student grades the strength of the hip abductors and verbalizes it to instructor.	☐	☐	☐
		Student asks patient if they had any pain during that motion. If yes, student asks patient to rate their pain and documents the results.	☐	☐	☐
	13	The student correctly measures **Hip Adduction MMT (against gravity)**:			
		Student verbalizes the primary muscles they are assessing: *(Adductor magnus, adductor longus, adductor brevis, pectineus, gracilis).*	☐	☐	☐
		Student places patient in a sidelying position with the tested limb resting on the table and the nontested limb supported by student in a position of 25 degrees of abduction.	☐	☐	☐
		Student instructs patient to adduct their hip through their full range of motion to ensure full active range of motion.	☐	☐	☐
		Student instructs patient to repeat that motion and then hold their leg in mid-range (15 degrees of adduction).	☐	☐	☐
		Student instructs patient to: *(Hold your leg in this position and do not let me push it down).*	☐	☐	☐
		Student applies moderate resistance proximal to the knee joint on the medial aspect of the thigh.	☐	☐	☐
		Student grades the strength of the hip adductors and verbalizes it to instructor.	☐	☐	☐
		Student asks patient if they had any pain during that motion. If yes, student asks patient to rate their pain and documents the results.	☐	☐	☐
	14	The student correctly measures **Hip Adduction MMT (gravity minimized)**:			
		Student places patient supine with the tested limb supported by the clinician in a slight amount of abduction and the nontested limb resting in 25 degrees of abduction.	☐	☐	☐
		Student instructs patient to adduct the hip through the range of motion. If no motion occurs at the joint, student palpates the muscle tendons to determine if there is a contraction.	☐	☐	☐
		Student grades the strength of the hip adductors and verbalizes it to instructor.	☐	☐	☐
		Student asks patient if they had any pain during that motion. If yes, student asks patient to rate their pain and documents the results.	☐	☐	☐

☐ = Critical Safety Element/Professionalism. If a student is unable to complete a flagged step without cueing, they will need to return at another time to redo the check-off. All other steps can be cued.

	15	The student correctly measures **Hip Internal Rotation MMT (against gravity)**:			
		Student verbalizes the primary muscles they are assessing: *(Gluteus medius, gluteus minimus, tensor fasciae latae).*	☐	☐	☐
		Student places patient in a seated position with the knees flexed over the edge of the table.	☐	☐	☐
		Student instructs patient to internally rotate their hip through their full range of motion to ensure full active range of motion.	☐	☐	☐
		Student instructs patient to repeat that motion and then hold their leg in mid-range (20–30 degrees of internal rotation).	☐	☐	☐
		Student applies stabilization to the distal thigh and the medial side of the knee joint.	☐	☐	☐
		Student instructs patient to: *(Hold your leg in this position and do not let me move it).*	☐	☐	☐
		Student applies moderate resistance to the lower leg just proximal to the lateral malleolus.	☐	☐	☐
		Student grades the strength of the hip internal rotators and verbalizes it to instructor.	☐	☐	☐
		Student asks patient if they had any pain during that motion. If yes, student asks patient to rate their pain and documents the results.	☐	☐	☐
	16	The student correctly measures **Hip Rotation MMT (gravity minimized)**:			
		Student places patient supine with the knees extended and the tested hip in slight external rotation.	☐	☐	☐
		Student instructs patient to internally rotate the hip through the range of motion. If no motion occurs at the joint, student palpates the muscle tendons to determine if there is a contraction.	☐	☐	☐
		Student grades the strength of the hip internal rotators and verbalizes it to instructor.	☐	☐	☐
		Student asks patient if they had any pain during that motion. If yes, student asks patient to rate their pain and documents the results.	☐	☐	☐
	17	The student correctly measures **Hip External Rotation MMT (against gravity)**:			
		Student verbalizes the primary muscles they are assessing: *(Obturator externus, obturator internus, piriformis, superior gemellus, inferior gemellus, quadratus femoris).*	☐	☐	☐
		Student places patient in a seated position with the knees flexed over the table's edge.	☐	☐	☐
		Student instructs patient to externally rotate their hip through their full range of motion to ensure full active range of motion.	☐	☐	☐
		Student instructs patient to repeat that motion and then hold their leg in mid-range (20–30 degrees of external rotation).	☐	☐	☐
		Student applies stabilization to the distal thigh and the lateral side of the knee joint.	☐	☐	☐
		Student instructs patient to: *(Hold your leg in this position and do not let me move it).*	☐	☐	☐
		Student applies moderate resistance to the lower leg just proximal to the medial malleolus.	☐	☐	☐
		Student grades the strength of the hip external rotators and verbalizes it to instructor.	☐	☐	☐
		Student asks patient if they had any pain during that motion. If yes, student asks patient to rate their pain and documents the results.	☐	☐	☐

☐ = Critical Safety Element/Professionalism. If a student is unable to complete a flagged step without cueing, they will need to return at another time to redo the check-off. All other steps can be cued.

	18	The student correctly measures **Hip External Rotation MMT (gravity minimized)**:			
		Student places patient supine with the knees extended and the tested hip in slight internal rotation.	☐	☐	☐
		Student instructs patient to externally rotate the hip through the range of motion. If no motion occurs at the joint, student palpates the muscle tendons to determine if there is a contraction.	☐	☐	☐
		Student grades the strength of the hip external rotators and verbalizes it to instructor.	☐	☐	☐
		Student asks patient if they had any pain during that motion. If yes, student asks patient to rate their pain and documents the results.	☐	☐	☐
Post-Skill	19	The student washes their hands post–skill performance:			
		Student removes all jewelry from their wrists and hands. Student turns the water to the preferred temperature and wets their hands. Student applies the soap to their hands and washes them with their hands pointed down. Student scrubs for 40–60 seconds and includes palm, between fingers, fingernails, and dorsum of hands. Student rinses hands with hands pointed down. Student dries their hands with a paper towel, uses a paper towel to turn off the water, and then disposes of the paper towel in the trash.	☐	☐	☐
	20	The student verbalizes that they will document their session in the note.	☐	☐	☐
Other	21 ⚐	The student has optimal body mechanics during performance of the skill.	☐	☐	☐
	22 ⚐	The student uses appropriate therapeutic touch.	☐	☐	☐
	23	The student is able to complete the check-off in the time allotted.	☐	☐	☐
Communication	24	The student uses language the patient can understand.	☐	☐	☐
	25	The student listens actively to the patient during the session.	☐	☐	☐
	26	The student ensures the patient understands instructions by having the patient teach back or demonstrate.	☐	☐	☐
	27 ⚐	The student demonstrates confidence and provides the patient with clear instruction and cueing.	☐	☐	☐

Peer Name (Printed)		**Peer Signature**		**Date of Peer Review**	
Instructor Name (Printed and Signature)	By signing this skills checklist, I am declaring this student competent in the skill described above.			**Date of Instructor Review**	

NOTES	

⚐ = Critical Safety Element/Professionalism. If a student is unable to complete a flagged step without cueing, they will need to return at another time to redo the check-off. All other steps can be cued.

Student Name: _____

Skill	Manual Muscle Testing: Knee			
Source	Van Ost L, Morogiello J. *Cram Session in Goniometry and Manual Muscle Testing: A Handbook for Students & Clinicians*. 2nd ed. SLACK Incorporated; 2023.	**Check When Completed**		
		Self	Peer	Instructor
Student Introduction and Consent	1 ⚑ The student introduces themself to the patient. Must include that they are a **student** PTA and list the school's name.	☐	☐	☐
	2 ⚑ The student verifies the patient's identity. Must use at least 2 patient identifiers (name, date of birth).	☐	☐	☐
	3 ⚑ The student gains consent: • Speaks with the patient about their status (acquires relevant information) • Educates the patient on intended data collection/intervention and goals for the session • Gains permission to perform said data collection/intervention	☐	☐	☐
Student, Patient, and Supply Preparation	4 ⚑ The student gathers supplies and prepares treatment area (cleans equipment, checks for safety hazards, ensures all equipment is functional and appropriate).	☐	☐	☐
	5 The student washes their hands:			
	Student removes all jewelry from their wrists and hands. Student turns the water to the preferred temperature and wets their hands. Student applies the soap to their hands and washes them with their hands pointed down. Student scrubs for 40–60 seconds and includes palm, between fingers, fingernails, and dorsum of hands. Student rinses hands with hands pointed down. Student dries their hands with a paper towel, uses a paper towel to turn off the water, and then disposes of the paper towel in the trash.	☐	☐	☐
	6 The student places the patient in the correct position for support, comfort, and access to body area necessary for data collection/intervention.	☐	☐	☐
Skill Performance	7 The student correctly measures **Knee Flexion MMT (against gravity):**			
	Student verbalizes the primary muscles they are assessing: *(Biceps femoris, semitendinosus, semimembranosus).*	☐	☐	☐
	Student places patient in a prone position with the tested hip in neutral rotation.	☐	☐	☐
	Student instructs patient to flex their knee through their full range of motion to ensure full active range of motion.	☐	☐	☐
	Student instructs patient to repeat that motion and then hold their leg in mid-range (45 degrees of flexion).	☐	☐	☐
	Student stabilizes the thigh against the table.	☐	☐	☐
	Student instructs patient to: *(Hold your leg in this position and do not let me push it down).*	☐	☐	☐
	Student applies moderate resistance just proximal to the posterior aspect of the ankle joint.	☐	☐	☐
	Student grades the strength of the knee flexors and verbalizes it to instructor.	☐	☐	☐
	Student asks patient if they had any pain during that motion. If yes, student asks patient to rate their pain and documents the results.	☐	☐	☐

⚑ = Critical Safety Element/Professionalism. If a student is unable to complete a flagged step without cueing, they will need to return at another time to redo the check-off. All other steps can be cued.

	8	The student correctly measures **Knee Flexion MMT (gravity minimized):**			
		Student places patient in sidelying with the tested limb on top and either supported by student or resting on a powder board. The lower limb is slightly flexed for stability.	☐	☐	☐
		Student instructs patient to flex the knee through the range of motion. If no motion occurs at the joint, student palpates the muscle tendons to determine if there is a contraction.	☐	☐	☐
		Student grades the strength of the knee flexors and verbalizes it to instructor.	☐	☐	☐
		Student asks patient if they had any pain during that motion. If yes, student asks patient to rate their pain and documents the results.	☐	☐	☐
	9	The student correctly measures **Knee Extension MMT (against gravity):**			
		Student verbalizes the primary muscles they are assessing: *(Rectus femoris, vastus intermedius, vastus medialis, vastus lateralis).*	☐	☐	☐
		Student places patient in a seated position with both knees flexed to 90 degrees and hanging freely over the edge of a table.	☐	☐	☐
		Student instructs patient to extend their knee through their full range of motion to ensure full active range of motion.	☐	☐	☐
		Student instructs patient to repeat that motion and then hold their leg in mid-range (45 degrees of flexion).	☐	☐	☐
		Student applies stabilization to the posterolateral aspect of the knee.	☐	☐	☐
		Student instructs patient to: *(Hold your leg in this position and do not let me move it).*	☐	☐	☐
		Student applies moderate resistance just proximal to the ankle joint on the anterior aspect of the lower leg.	☐	☐	☐
		Student grades the strength of the knee extensors and verbalizes it to instructor.	☐	☐	☐
		Student asks patient if they had any pain during that motion. If yes, student asks patient to rate their pain and documents the results.	☐	☐	☐
	10	The student correctly measures **Knee Extension MMT (gravity minimized):**			
		Student places patient in sidelying with the tested limb on top, resting on a powder board with the knee flexed to 90 degrees. The bottom knee should be slightly flexed for stability.	☐	☐	☐
		Student instructs patient to extend the knee through the range of motion. If no motion occurs at the joint, student palpates the muscle tendons to determine if there is a contraction.	☐	☐	☐
		Student grades the strength of the knee extensors and verbalizes it to instructor.	☐	☐	☐
		Student asks patient if they had any pain during that motion. If yes, student asks patient to rate their pain and documents the results.	☐	☐	☐
Post-Skill	11	The student washes their hands post–skill performance:			
		Student removes all jewelry from their wrists and hands. Student turns the water to the preferred temperature and wets their hands. Student applies the soap to their hands and washes them with their hands pointed down. Student scrubs for 40–60 seconds and includes palm, between fingers, fingernails, and dorsum of hands. Student rinses hands with hands pointed down. Student dries their hands with a paper towel, uses a paper towel to turn off the water, and then disposes of the paper towel in the trash.	☐	☐	☐
	12	The student verbalizes that they will document their session in the note.	☐	☐	☐
Other	13 ⚑	The student has optimal body mechanics during performance of the skill.	☐	☐	☐
	14 ⚑	The student uses appropriate therapeutic touch.	☐	☐	☐
	15	The student is able to complete the check-off in the time allotted.	☐	☐	☐

⚑ = Critical Safety Element/Professionalism. If a student is unable to complete a flagged step without cueing, they will need to return at another time to redo the check-off. All other steps can be cued.

Communication	16	The student uses language the patient can understand.	☐	☐	☐
	17	The student listens actively to the patient during the session.	☐	☐	☐
	18	The student ensures the patient understands instructions by having the patient teach back or demonstrate.	☐	☐	☐
	19 ⚐	The student demonstrates confidence and provides the patient with clear instruction and cueing.	☐	☐	☐

Peer Name (Printed)		Peer Signature		Date of Peer Review	
Instructor Name (Printed and Signature)	By signing this skills checklist, I am declaring this student competent in the skill described above.			Date of Instructor Review	
NOTES					

⚐ = Critical Safety Element/Professionalism. If a student is unable to complete a flagged step without cueing, they will need to return at another time to redo the check-off. All other steps can be cued.

Student Name: _____

Skill		Manual Muscle Testing: Ankle			
Source		Van Ost L, Morogiello J. *Cram Session in Goniometry and Manual Muscle Testing: A Handbook for Students & Clinicians*. 2nd ed. SLACK Incorporated; 2023.	Check When Completed		
			Self	Peer	Instructor
Student Introduction and Consent	1 ⚑	The student introduces themself to the patient. Must include that they are a **student** PTA and list the school's name.	☐	☐	☐
	2 ⚑	The student verifies the patient's identity. Must use at least 2 patient identifiers (name, date of birth).	☐	☐	☐
	3 ⚑	The student gains consent: • Speaks with the patient about their status (acquires relevant information) • Educates the patient on intended data collection/intervention and goals for the session • Gains permission to perform said data collection/intervention	☐	☐	☐
Student, Patient, and Supply Preparation	4 ⚑	The student gathers supplies and prepares treatment area (cleans equipment, checks for safety hazards, ensures all equipment is functional and appropriate).	☐	☐	☐
	5	The student washes their hands:			
		Student removes all jewelry from their wrists and hands. Student turns the water to the preferred temperature and wets their hands. Student applies the soap to their hands and washes them with their hands pointed down. Student scrubs for 40–60 seconds and includes palm, between fingers, fingernails, and dorsum of hands. Student rinses hands with hands pointed down. Student dries their hands with a paper towel, uses a paper towel to turn off the water, and then disposes of the paper towel in the trash.	☐	☐	☐
	6	The student places the patient in the correct position for support, comfort, and access to body area necessary for data collection/intervention.	☐	☐	☐
Skill Performance	7	The student correctly measures **Ankle Dorsiflexion/Inversion MMT (against gravity):**			
		Student verbalizes the primary muscle they are assessing: *(Tibialis anterior)*.	☐	☐	☐
		Student places patient in a seated position with the knee flexed over the edge of a table with the ankle/foot in a relaxed position.	☐	☐	☐
		Student instructs patient to bring their foot up and in (combined dorsiflexion and inversion) through their full range of motion to ensure full active range of motion.	☐	☐	☐
		Student instructs patient to repeat that motion and then hold their ankle in mid-range.	☐	☐	☐
		Student stabilizes the lower leg.	☐	☐	☐
		Student instructs patient to: *(Hold your ankle in this position and do not let me move it).*	☐	☐	☐
		Student applies moderate resistance to the medial/dorsal surface of the forefoot into plantarflexion/eversion.	☐	☐	☐
		Student grades the strength of the anterior tibialis and verbalizes it to instructor.	☐	☐	☐
		Student asks patient if they had any pain during that motion. If yes, student asks patient to rate their pain and documents the results.	☐	☐	☐

⚑ = Critical Safety Element/Professionalism. If a student is unable to complete a flagged step without cueing, they will need to return at another time to redo the check-off. All other steps can be cued.

	8	The student correctly measures **Ankle Dorsiflexion/Inversion MMT (gravity minimized):**			
		Student places patient in sidelying with the tested limb/ankle on top resting on a powder board or smooth surface.	☐	☐	☐
		Student instructs patient to dorsiflex and invert the ankle through the range of motion. If no motion occurs at the joint, student palpates the muscle tendons to determine if there is a contraction.	☐	☐	☐
		Student grades the strength of the tibialis anterior and verbalizes it to instructor.	☐	☐	☐
		Student asks patient if they had any pain during that motion. If yes, student asks patient to rate their pain and documents the results.	☐	☐	☐
	9	The student correctly measures **Ankle Inversion MMT (against gravity):**			
		Student verbalizes the primary muscle they are assessing: *(Tibialis posterior).*	☐	☐	☐
		Student places patient in sidelying with the tested foot and ankle over the edge of a table.	☐	☐	☐
		Student instructs patient to invert their ankle through their full range of motion to ensure full active range of motion.	☐	☐	☐
		Student instructs patient to repeat that motion and then hold their ankle in mid-range.	☐	☐	☐
		Student applies stabilization to the lower limb.	☐	☐	☐
		Student instructs patient to: *(Hold your ankle in this position and do not let me move it).*	☐	☐	☐
		Student applies moderate resistance to the medial border of the forefoot into eversion and dorsiflexion.	☐	☐	☐
		Student grades the strength of the ankle invertors and verbalizes it to instructor.	☐	☐	☐
		Student asks patient if they had any pain during that motion. If yes, student asks patient to rate their pain and documents the results.	☐	☐	☐
	10	The student correctly measures **Ankle Inversion MMT (gravity minimized):**			
		Student places patient in supine with the tested foot/ankle over the edge of a table.	☐	☐	☐
		Student instructs patient to invert the ankle through the range of motion. If no motion occurs at the joint, student palpates the muscle tendons to determine if there is a contraction.	☐	☐	☐
		Student grades the strength of the ankle invertors and verbalizes it to instructor.	☐	☐	☐
		Student asks patient if they had any pain during that motion. If yes, student asks patient to rate their pain and documents the results.	☐	☐	☐
	11	The student correctly measures **Ankle Eversion MMT (against gravity):**			
		Student verbalizes the primary muscles they are assessing: *(Peroneus longus, peroneus brevis, peroneus tertius).*	☐	☐	☐
		Student places patient in sidelying with the tested foot and ankle over the edge of a table.	☐	☐	☐
		Student instructs patient to evert their ankle through their full range of motion to ensure full active range of motion.	☐	☐	☐
		Student instructs patient to repeat that motion and then hold their ankle in mid-range.	☐	☐	☐
		Student applies stabilization to the lower limb.	☐	☐	☐
		Student instructs patient to: *(Hold your ankle in this position and do not let me move it).*	☐	☐	☐
		Student applies moderate resistance to the lateral border of the forefoot into inversion and plantarflexion.	☐	☐	☐
		Student grades the strength of the ankle evertors and verbalizes it to instructor.	☐	☐	☐
		Student asks patient if they had any pain during that motion. If yes, student asks patient to rate their pain and documents the results.	☐	☐	☐

☐ = Critical Safety Element/Professionalism. If a student is unable to complete a flagged step without cueing, they will need to return at another time to redo the check-off. All other steps can be cued.

	12	The student correctly measures **Ankle Eversion MMT (gravity minimized):**			
		Student places patient in supine with the tested foot/ankle over the edge of a table.	☐	☐	☐
		Student instructs patient to evert the ankle through the range of motion. If no motion occurs at the joint, student palpates the muscle tendons to determine if there is a contraction.	☐	☐	☐
		Student grades the strength of the ankle evertors and verbalizes it to instructor.	☐	☐	☐
		Student asks patient if they had any pain during that motion. If yes, student asks patient to rate their pain and documents the results.	☐	☐	☐
	13	The student correctly measures **Ankle Plantarflexion MMT (against gravity):**			
		Student verbalizes the primary muscles they are assessing: *(Gastrocnemius, plantaris, soleus).*	☐	☐	☐
		Student places patient in single leg standing on the tested limb with the knee in maximal extension. The opposite foot should be off the floor and patient should balance themself with 1–2 fingers on a tabletop or countertop.	☐	☐	☐
		Student instructs patient to perform a heel raise through their full range of motion to ensure full active range of motion and good form.	☐	☐	☐
		Student instructs patient to: *(Repeat this as many times as you can until I tell you to stop).*	☐	☐	☐
		Student stops patient if/when they have decreased motion or form is no longer good.	☐	☐	☐
		Student grades the strength of the plantarflexors and verbalizes it to instructor: *(25 heel raises = 5/5* *10–24 heel raises = 4/5* *1–9 heel raises = 3/5).*	☐	☐	☐
		Student asks patient if they had any pain during that motion. If yes, student asks patient to rate their pain and documents the results.	☐	☐	☐
	14	The student correctly measures **Ankle Plantarflexion MMT (gravity minimized):**			
		Student places patient in prone with the tested foot/ankle off the edge of a table.	☐	☐	☐
		Student instructs patient to plantarflex the ankle through the range of motion. If no motion occurs at the joint, student palpates the muscle tendons to determine if there is a contraction.	☐	☐	☐
		Student grades the strength of the ankle plantarflexors and verbalizes it to instructor.	☐	☐	☐
		Student asks patient if they had any pain during that motion. If yes, student asks patient to rate their pain and documents the results.	☐	☐	☐
Post-Skill	15	The student washes their hands post–skill performance:			
		Student removes all jewelry from their wrists and hands. Student turns the water to the preferred temperature and wets their hands. Student applies the soap to their hands and washes them with their hands pointed down. Student scrubs for 40–60 seconds and includes palm, between fingers, fingernails, and dorsum of hands. Student rinses hands with hands pointed down. Student dries their hands with a paper towel, uses a paper towel to turn off the water, and then disposes of the paper towel in the trash.	☐	☐	☐
	16	The student verbalizes that they will document their session in the note.	☐	☐	☐
Other	17 ⚑	The student has optimal body mechanics during performance of the skill.	☐	☐	☐
	18 ⚑	The student uses appropriate therapeutic touch.	☐	☐	☐
	19	The student is able to complete the check-off in the time allotted.	☐	☐	☐

⚑ = Critical Safety Element/Professionalism. If a student is unable to complete a flagged step without cueing, they will need to return at another time to redo the check-off. All other steps can be cued.

Communication	20	The student uses language the patient can understand.	☐	☐	☐
	21	The student listens actively to the patient during the session.	☐	☐	☐
	22	The student ensures the patient understands instructions by having the patient teach back or demonstrate.	☐	☐	☐
	23 ⚑	The student demonstrates confidence and provides the patient with clear instruction and cueing.	☐	☐	☐

Peer Name (Printed)		**Peer Signature**		**Date of Peer Review**	
Instructor Name (Printed and Signature)	By signing this skills checklist, I am declaring this student competent in the skill described above.			**Date of Instructor Review**	
NOTES					

⚑ = Critical Safety Element/Professionalism. If a student is unable to complete a flagged step without cueing, they will need to return at another time to redo the check-off. All other steps can be cued.

Chapter 6

Muscle Length Testing

Larson T. *Entry-Level Skill Checklists for*
Physical Therapist Assistant Students (pp 89-96).
© 2023 Taylor & Francis Group.

Student Name: _____

Skill		Muscle Length Testing: Upper Quarter			
Source		Physical Therapy. Education. Redefined. PhysioU. Accessed September 14, 2022. https://www.physiou.health/	Check When Completed		
			Self	Peer	Instructor
Student Introduction and Consent	1 ⚑	The student introduces themself to the patient. Must include that they are a **student** PTA and list the school's name.	☐	☐	☐
	2 ⚑	The student verifies the patient's identity. Must use at least 2 patient identifiers (name, date of birth).	☐	☐	☐
	3 ⚑	The student gains consent: • Speaks with the patient about their status (acquires relevant information) • Educates the patient on intended data collection/intervention and goals for the session • Gains permission to perform said data collection/intervention	☐	☐	☐
Student, Patient, and Supply Preparation	4 ⚑	The student gathers supplies and prepares treatment area (cleans equipment, checks for safety hazards, ensures all equipment is functional and appropriate).	☐	☐	☐
	5	The student washes their hands:			
		Student removes all jewelry from their wrists and hands. Student turns the water to the preferred temperature and wets their hands. Student applies the soap to their hands and washes them with their hands pointed down. Student scrubs for 40–60 seconds and includes palm, between fingers, fingernails, and dorsum of hands. Student rinses hands with hands pointed down. Student dries their hands with a paper towel, uses a paper towel to turn off the water, and then disposes of the paper towel in the trash.	☐	☐	☐
	6	The student places the patient in the correct position for support, comfort, and access to body area necessary for data collection/intervention.	☐	☐	☐
Skill Performance	7	The student correctly measures **Pectoralis Major Muscle Length**:			
		Student places patient in a supine position.	☐	☐	☐
		Student instructs patient to place their uninvolved arm across their chest, creating a barrier.	☐	☐	☐
		Student uses their own forearm on patients uninvolved arm to stabilize patient's thorax to the table.	☐	☐	☐
		Student assesses the length of the sternal fibers by passively taking patient's shoulder into 120 degrees of abduction and full external rotation while letting the arm fall toward the floor.	☐	☐	☐
		Student verbalizes to instructor the results of the length test: *(A normal test is to be able to reach the height of the table).*	☐	☐	☐
		Student assesses the length of the clavicular fibers passively taking patient's arm to 90 degrees of abduction and letting the arm fall toward the floor.	☐	☐	☐
		Student verbalizes to instructor the results of the length test: *(A normal test is to be able to reach the height of the table).*	☐	☐	☐
		Repeat on the opposite limb.	☐	☐	☐
		Student asks patient if they had any pain during that motion. If yes, student asks patient to rate their pain and documents the results.	☐	☐	☐
	8	The student correctly measures **Pectoralis Minor Muscle Length**:			
		Student places patient in a supine position.	☐	☐	☐
		Student palpates acromion and measures the distance between the most posterior aspect of acromion and the table with a tape measure.	☐	☐	☐
		Student verbalizes to instructor the results of the length test: *(A normal test is 1 inch or less).*	☐	☐	☐

⚑ = Critical Safety Element/Professionalism. If a student is unable to complete a flagged step without cueing, they will need to return at another time to redo the check-off. All other steps can be cued.

	9	The student correctly measures **Subscapularis Muscle Length**:			
		Student places patient in a supine position.	☐	☐	☐
		Student passively measures patient's degree of shoulder external rotation with arm by their side (0 degrees of abduction) AND with their arm at 90 degrees of abduction.	☐	☐	☐
		Student verbalizes to instructor the results of the length test: *(A positive test for a short subscapularis muscle occurs when there is limited range at patient's side and full range at 90 degrees of abduction).*	☐	☐	☐
		Student asks patient if they had any pain during that motion. If yes, student asks patient to rate their pain and documents the results.	☐	☐	☐
	10	The student correctly measures **Teres Major Muscle Length**:			
		Student places patient in a supine position.	☐	☐	☐
		Student moves patient's shoulder passively into flexion while maintaining full external rotation and using the other hand to stabilize the scapula to prevent it from moving past the midaxillary line.	☐	☐	☐
		Student moves patient's arm into full flexion until an end feel is felt.	☐	☐	☐
		Student then internally rotates the humerus and attempts to move patient into more flexion.	☐	☐	☐
		Student verbalizes to instructor the results of the length test: *(A positive test is when the therapist internally rotates the humerus, and patient can go much farther into shoulder flexion).*	☐	☐	☐
		Student asks patient if they had any pain during that motion. If yes, student asks patient to rate their pain and documents the results.	☐	☐	☐
	11	The student correctly measures **Biceps Brachii Muscle Length**:			
		Student places patient in a supine position with elbow in 90 degrees of flexion and neutral rotation.	☐	☐	☐
		Student instructs patient to hang the arm off the edge of the table, maintaining elbow flexion.	☐	☐	☐
		Student passively assesses elbow extension with forearm fully pronated to end range of motion, maintaining 90 degrees of shoulder extension: *(Stationary arm = acromion process Axis = lateral epicondyle Movement arm = radial styloid process).*	☐	☐	☐
		Student verbalizes to instructor the results of the length test: *(A normal test reaches 0–compared to opposite limb).*	☐	☐	☐
		Student asks patient if they had any pain during that motion. If yes, student asks patient to rate their pain and documents the results.	☐	☐	☐
	12	The student correctly measures **Triceps Brachii Muscle Length**:			
		Student places patient in supine with full shoulder flexion.	☐	☐	☐
		Student instructs patient to flex their elbow, maintaining shoulder flexion.	☐	☐	☐
		Student passively assesses elbow flexion with forearm fully supinated to end range of motion, maintaining full shoulder flexion: *(Stationary arm = acromion process Axis = lateral epicondyle Movement arm = radial styloid process).*	☐	☐	☐
		Student verbalizes to instructor the results of the length test: *(Compare to opposite limb).*	☐	☐	☐
		Student asks patient if they had any pain during that motion. If yes, student asks patient to rate their pain and documents the results.	☐	☐	☐

☐ = Critical Safety Element/Professionalism. If a student is unable to complete a flagged step without cueing, they will need to return at another time to redo the check-off. All other steps can be cued.

	13	The student correctly measures **Wrist Flexors Muscle Length**:			
		Student places patient in seated position with shoulder flexed to 90 degrees, elbow fully extended, forearm in pronation and supported on table.	☐	☐	☐
		Student passively extends the wrist, pushing through the fingers to end range of motion.	☐	☐	☐
		Student passively measures wrist extension in this position: *(Stationary arm = ulnar styloid process to the olecranon* *Axis = lateral triquetrum* *Movement arm = parallel with 5th metacarpal).*	☐	☐	☐
		Student verbalizes to instructor the results of the length test: *(Compare to opposite limb).*	☐	☐	☐
		Student asks patient if they had any pain during that motion. If yes, student asks patient to rate their pain and documents the results.	☐	☐	☐
	14	The student correctly measures **Wrist Extensors Muscle Length**:			
		Student places patient in seated position with shoulder flexed to 90 degrees, elbow fully extended, forearm in pronation and supported on table, wrist hanging off table.	☐	☐	☐
		Student instructs patient to grasp the thumb with the fingers to make a fist.	☐	☐	☐
		Student passively flexes the wrist to end range of motion.	☐	☐	☐
		Student passively measures wrist flexion in this position: *(Stationary arm = ulnar styloid process to the olecranon* *Axis = lateral triquetrum* *Movement arm = parallel with 5th metacarpal).*	☐	☐	☐
		Student verbalizes to instructor the results of the length test: *(Compare to opposite limb).*	☐	☐	☐
		Student asks patient if they had any pain during that motion. If yes, student asks patient to rate their pain and documents the results.	☐	☐	☐
Post-Skill	15	The student washes their hands post–skill performance:			
		Student removes all jewelry from their wrists and hands. Student turns the water to the preferred temperature and wets their hands. Student applies the soap to their hands and washes them with their hands pointed down. Student scrubs for 40–60 seconds and includes palm, between fingers, fingernails, and dorsum of hands. Student rinses hands with hands pointed down. Student dries their hands with a paper towel, uses a paper towel to turn off the water, and then disposes of the paper towel in the trash.	☐	☐	☐
	16	The student verbalizes that they will document their session in the note.	☐	☐	☐
Other	17 ⚑	The student has optimal body mechanics during performance of the skill.	☐	☐	☐
	18 ⚑	The student uses appropriate therapeutic touch.	☐	☐	☐
	19	The student is able to complete the check-off in the time allotted.	☐	☐	☐

⚑ = Critical Safety Element/Professionalism. If a student is unable to complete a flagged step without cueing, they will need to return at another time to redo the check-off. All other steps can be cued.

Communication	20	The student uses language the patient can understand.	☐	☐	☐
	21	The student listens actively to the patient during the session.	☐	☐	☐
	22	The student ensures the patient understands instructions by having the patient teach back or demonstrate.	☐	☐	☐
	23 ⚑	The student demonstrates confidence and provides the patient with clear instruction and cueing.	☐	☐	☐

Peer Name (Printed)		**Peer Signature**		**Date of Peer Review**	
Instructor Name (Printed and Signature)	By signing this skills checklist, I am declaring this student competent in the skill described above.			**Date of Instructor Review**	

NOTES	

⚑ = Critical Safety Element/Professionalism. If a student is unable to complete a flagged step without cueing, they will need to return at another time to redo the check-off. All other steps can be cued.

Student Name: _____

Skill		Muscle Length Testing: Lower Quarter			
Source		Physical Therapy. Education. Redefined. PhysioU. Accessed September 14, 2022. https://www.physiou.health/	**Check When Completed**		
			Self	Peer	Instructor
Student Introduction and Consent	1 ⚑	The student introduces themself to the patient. Must include that they are a **student** PTA and list the school's name.	☐	☐	☐
	2 ⚑	The student verifies the patient's identity. Must use at least 2 patient identifiers (name, date of birth).	☐	☐	☐
	3 ⚑	The student gains consent: • Speaks with the patient about their status (acquires relevant information) • Educates the patient on intended data collection/intervention and goals for the session • Gains permission to perform said data collection/intervention	☐	☐	☐
Student, Patient, and Supply Preparation	4 ⚑	The student gathers supplies and prepares treatment area (cleans equipment, checks for safety hazards, ensures all equipment is functional and appropriate).	☐	☐	☐
	5	The student washes their hands:			
		Student removes all jewelry from their wrists and hands. Student turns the water to the preferred temperature and wets their hands. Student applies the soap to their hands and washes them with their hands pointed down. Student scrubs for 40–60 seconds and includes palm, between fingers, fingernails, and dorsum of hands. Student rinses hands with hands pointed down. Student dries their hands with a paper towel, uses a paper towel to turn off the water, and then disposes of the paper towel in the trash.	☐	☐	☐
	6	The student places the patient in the correct position for support, comfort, and access to body area necessary for data collection/intervention.	☐	☐	☐
Skill Performance	7	The student correctly measures **Hip Flexor Muscle Length (Thomas Test)**:			
		Student places patient in a seated position at the edge of the table, holding one leg under thigh with both hands.	☐	☐	☐
		Student helps lower patient onto their back and lifts the opposite leg into hip flexion. Patient can hold this leg up with their hands or student can support the foot on their lateral trunk.	☐	☐	☐
		Student lowers the tested leg down, while feeling the contralateral ASIS, to assess for any movement of the pelvis and to feel for true length of hip flexors.	☐	☐	☐
		Student verbalizes to instructor the results of the length test: *(Normal: hip to 0 degrees, knee to 90 degrees, neutral femoral position in line with the hip, neutral pelvis and lumbar spine [no movement noted]).*	☐	☐	☐
		Student asks patient if they had any pain during that motion. If yes, student asks patient to rate their pain and documents the results.	☐	☐	☐

⚑ = Critical Safety Element/Professionalism. If a student is unable to complete a flagged step without cueing, they will need to return at another time to redo the check-off. All other steps can be cued.

	8	The student correctly measures **Rectus Femoris Muscle Length (Ely's Test):**			
		Student places patient in a prone position.	☐	☐	☐
		Student flexes patient's knee to the end of the range of motion determined by resistance to movement, increased hip flexion, anterior pelvic tilt, or lumbar spine extension.	☐	☐	☐
		Student passively assesses knee flexion in this position: *(Stationary arm = lateral midline of femur to greater trochanter Axis = lateral epicondyle of the femur Movement arm = lateral midline of fibula to lateral malleolus).*	☐	☐	☐
		Student verbalizes to instructor the results of the length test: *(If the knee can be flexed to at least 90 degrees with the hip in the neutral position, the length of the rectus femoris is considered normal).*	☐	☐	☐
		Student asks patient if they had any pain during that motion. If yes, student asks patient to rate their pain and documents the results.	☐	☐	☐
	9	The student correctly measures **Hamstring Muscle Length:**			
		Student places patient in a supine position.	☐	☐	☐
		Student passively flexes patient hip to the end of the range of motion, determined by resistance to movement, knee flexion, posterior pelvic tilt, or lumbar spine flexion.	☐	☐	☐
		Student passively assesses hip flexion in this position: *(Stationary arm = lateral midline of pelvis Axis = greater trochanter Movement arm = midline of lateral femur to lateral epicondyle of ipsilateral knee).*	☐	☐	☐
		Student verbalizes to instructor the results of the length test: *(70–80 degrees of hip flexion is considered normal).*	☐	☐	☐
		Student asks patient if they had any pain during that motion. If yes, student asks patient to rate their pain and documents the results.	☐	☐	☐
	10	The student correctly measures **Piriformis Muscle Length:**			
		Student places patient in a supine position.	☐	☐	☐
		Student moves the patient's hip into flexion above 90 degrees and adds external rotation by grasping the ankle.	☐	☐	☐
		Student moves patient's hip into adduction while maintaining the flexion and external rotation until an end feel is felt.	☐	☐	☐
		Student verbalizes to instructor the results of the length test: *(Compare to opposite limb).*	☐	☐	☐
		Student asks patient if they had any pain during that motion. If yes, student asks patient to rate their pain and documents the results.	☐	☐	☐
	11	The student correctly measures **Gastrocnemius Muscle Length:**			
		Student places patient in a prone position with knee extended to 0 degrees and ankle hanging off table.	☐	☐	☐
		Student finds subtalar neutral and passively dorsiflexes ankle to end range of motion, determined by resistance to motion or knee extension.	☐	☐	☐
		Student passively assesses ankle dorsiflexion in this position: *(Stationary arm = lateral midline of fibula to lateral epicondyle of femur Axis = lateral malleolus Movement arm = parallel to 5th metatarsal).*	☐	☐	☐
		Student verbalizes to instructor the results of the length test: *(10 degrees of dorsiflexion in this position is considered normal).*	☐	☐	☐
		Student asks patient if they had any pain during that motion. If yes, student asks patient to rate their pain and documents the results.	☐	☐	☐

⚑ = Critical Safety Element/Professionalism. If a student is unable to complete a flagged step without cueing, they will need to return at another time to redo the check-off. All other steps can be cued.

Post-Skill	12	The student washes their hands post–skill performance:			
		Student removes all jewelry from their wrists and hands. Student turns the water to the preferred temperature and wets their hands. Student applies the soap to their hands and washes them with their hands pointed down. Student scrubs for 40–60 seconds and includes palm, between fingers, fingernails, and dorsum of hands. Student rinses hands with hands pointed down. Student dries their hands with a paper towel, uses a paper towel to turn off the water, and then disposes of the paper towel in the trash.	☐	☐	☐
	13	The student verbalizes that they will document their session in the note.	☐	☐	☐
Other	14 ⚐	The student has optimal body mechanics during performance of the skill.	☐	☐	☐
	15 ⚐	The student uses appropriate therapeutic touch.	☐	☐	☐
	16	The student is able to complete the check-off in the time allotted.	☐	☐	☐
Communication	17	The student uses language the patient can understand.	☐	☐	☐
	18	The student listens actively to the patient during the session.	☐	☐	☐
	19	The student ensures the patient understands instructions by having the patient teach back or demonstrate.	☐	☐	☐
	20 ⚐	The student demonstrates confidence and provides the patient with clear instruction and cueing.	☐	☐	☐

Peer Name (Printed)		**Peer Signature**		**Date of Peer Review**
Instructor Name (Printed and Signature)	By signing this skills checklist, I am declaring this student competent in the skill described above.			**Date of Instructor Review**
NOTES				

⚐ = Critical Safety Element/Professionalism. If a student is unable to complete a flagged step without cueing, they will need to return at another time to redo the check-off. All other steps can be cued.

Chapter 7

Posture

Larson T. *Entry-Level Skill Checklists for Physical Therapist Assistant Students* (pp 97-99).
© 2023 Taylor & Francis Group.

Student Name: _____

Skill		Posture			
Source		Klaczak Kopack J, Cascardi KA. *Principles of Therapeutic Exercise for the Physical Therapist Assistant.* SLACK Incorporated; 2023.	**Check When Completed**		
			Self	Peer	Instructor
Student Introduction and Consent	1 ⚑	The student introduces themself to the patient. Must include that they are a **student** PTA and list the school's name.	☐	☐	☐
	2 ⚑	The student verifies the patient's identity. Must use at least 2 patient identifiers (name, date of birth).	☐	☐	☐
	3 ⚑	The student gains consent: • Speaks with the patient about their status (acquires relevant information) • Educates the patient on intended data collection/intervention and goals for the session • Gains permission to perform said data collection/intervention	☐	☐	☐
Student, Patient, and Supply Preparation	4 ⚑	The student gathers supplies and prepares treatment area (cleans equipment, checks for safety hazards, ensures all equipment is functional and appropriate).	☐	☐	☐
	5	The student washes their hands:			
		Student removes all jewelry from their wrists and hands. Student turns the water to the preferred temperature and wets their hands. Student applies the soap to their hands and washes them with their hands pointed down. Student scrubs for 40–60 seconds and includes palm, between fingers, fingernails, and dorsum of hands. Student rinses hands with hands pointed down. Student dries their hands with a paper towel, uses a paper towel to turn off the water, and then disposes of the paper towel in the trash.	☐	☐	☐
	6	The student places the patient in the correct position for support, comfort, and access to body area necessary for data collection/intervention.	☐	☐	☐
Skill Performance	7	The student correctly performs **Postural Assessment**:			
		Student assesses posture in standing from lateral view: The plumb line should be aligned just anteriorly to the lateral malleolus. The line of gravity should pass through the external auditory meatus, fall slightly posterior to the cervical spine, slightly anterior to the thoracic spine, and through the vertebral bodies of the lumbar spine. It should bisect the humerus, pass through the greater trochanter, and fall just posterior to the patella but just anterior to the knee joint.	☐	☐	☐
		Student assesses posture in standing from posterior view: The line of gravity should divide the head in equal halves, pass straight down between the scapulae along the vertebral column. It should also pass through the gluteal cleft and be of equal distance between the PSISs, the medial knee joints, and medial malleoli. The shoulders should be fairly level. Both PSISs and gluteal folds should also be level.	☐	☐	☐
		Student assesses posture in standing from anterior view: The line of gravity should pass through the middle of the forehead, nose, and chin, along the sternum through the umbilicus and equidistant between the ASISs, medial knee joints, and medial malleoli. The tibial tubercles should be facing forward, and the tibia should be vertical and foot in subtalar neutral.	☐	☐	☐
Post-Skill	8	The student washes their hands post–skill performance:			
		Student removes all jewelry from their wrists and hands. Student turns the water to the preferred temperature and wets their hands. Student applies the soap to their hands and washes them with their hands pointed down. Student scrubs for 40–60 seconds and includes palm, between fingers, fingernails, and dorsum of hands. Student rinses hands with hands pointed down. Student dries their hands with a paper towel, uses a paper towel to turn off the water, and then disposes of the paper towel in the trash.	☐	☐	☐
	9	The student verbalizes that they will document their session in the note.	☐	☐	☐

⚑ = Critical Safety Element/Professionalism. If a student is unable to complete a flagged step without cueing, they will need to return at another time to redo the check-off. All other steps can be cued.

	10 ⚑	The student has optimal body mechanics during performance of the skill.	☐	☐	☐
Other	11 ⚑	The student uses appropriate therapeutic touch.	☐	☐	☐
	12	The student is able to complete the check-off in the time allotted.	☐	☐	☐
Communication	13	The student uses language the patient can understand.	☐	☐	☐
	14	The student listens actively to the patient during the session.	☐	☐	☐
	15	The student ensures the patient understands instructions by having the patient teach back or demonstrate.	☐	☐	☐
	16 ⚑	The student demonstrates confidence and provides the patient with clear instruction and cueing.	☐	☐	☐

Peer Name (Printed)		Peer Signature		Date of Peer Review	
Instructor Name (Printed and Signature)	By signing this skills checklist, I am declaring this student competent in the skill described above.			Date of Instructor Review	
NOTES					

⚑ = Critical Safety Element/Professionalism. If a student is unable to complete a flagged step without cueing, they will need to return at another time to redo the check-off. All other steps can be cued.

Chapter 8
Wheelchair Measurement

Larson T. *Entry-Level Skill Checklists for
Physical Therapist Assistant Students* (pp 101-103).
© 2023 Taylor & Francis Group.

Student Name: _____

Skill		Wheelchair Measurement				
Source		Memolo J. *Procedures and Patient Care for the Physical Therapist Assistant.* SLACK Incorporated; 2019.	**Check When Completed**			
				Self	Peer	Instructor
Student Introduction and Consent	1 ⚑	The student introduces themself to the patient. Must include that they are a **student** PTA and list the school's name.		☐	☐	☐
	2 ⚑	The student verifies the patient's identity. Must use at least 2 patient identifiers (name, date of birth).		☐	☐	☐
	3 ⚑	The student gains consent: <ul><li>Speaks with the patient about their status (acquires relevant information)</li><li>Educates the patient on intended data collection/intervention and goals for the session</li><li>Gains permission to perform said data collection/intervention</li></ul>		☐	☐	☐
Student, Patient, and Supply Preparation	4 ⚑	The student gathers supplies and prepares treatment area (cleans equipment, checks for safety hazards, ensures all equipment is functional and appropriate).		☐	☐	☐
	5	The student washes their hands:				
		Student removes all jewelry from their wrists and hands. Student turns the water to the preferred temperature and wets their hands. Student applies the soap to their hands and washes them with their hands pointed down. Student scrubs for 40–60 seconds and includes palm, between fingers, fingernails, and dorsum of hands. Student rinses hands with hands pointed down. Student dries their hands with a paper towel, uses a paper towel to turn off the water, and then disposes of the paper towel in the trash.		☐	☐	☐
	6	The student positions patient in the correct position for support, comfort, and access to body area necessary for data collection/intervention. The patient should be sitting on a firm surface (not in wheelchair).		☐	☐	☐
Skill Performance	7	The student correctly measures **Seat Height/Leg Length**:				
		Student measures from patient's heel to popliteal fold and adds 2 inches to allow clearance of footrest. Student must consider the height of the seat cushion if one is present.		☐	☐	☐
	8	The student correctly measures **Seat Depth**:				
		Student measures from patient's posterior buttock along the lateral thigh to the popliteal fold and subtracts 2 inches to avoid pressure from seat on popliteal space.		☐	☐	☐
	9	The student correctly measures **Seat Width**:				
		Student measures the widest aspect of buttocks/hips and adds 2 inches to allow for clearance of hips in chair.		☐	☐	☐
	10	The student correctly measures **Back Height**:				
		Student measures from the seat of the chair to the floor of the axilla with patient's shoulder flexed at 90 degrees and subtracts 4 inches to allow the height to be below the inferior angle of the scapulae. Student must consider the height of the seat cushion if one is present.		☐	☐	☐
	11	The student correctly measures **Armrest Height**:				
		Student measures from the seat of the chair to the olecranon process with patient's elbow flexed at 90 degrees and adds 1 inch to allow correct posture and postural changes while seated. Student must consider the height of the seat cushion if one is present.		☐	☐	☐

⚑ = Critical Safety Element/Professionalism. If a student is unable to complete a flagged step without cueing, they will need to return at another time to redo the check-off. All other steps can be cued.

Post-Skill	12	The student washes their hands post–skill performance:			
		Student removes all jewelry from their wrists and hands. Student turns the water to the preferred temperature and wets their hands. Student applies the soap to their hands and washes them with their hands pointed down. Student scrubs for 40–60 seconds and includes palm, between fingers, fingernails, and dorsum of hands. Student rinses hands with hands pointed down. Student dries their hands with a paper towel, uses a paper towel to turn off the water, and then disposes of the paper towel in the trash.	☐	☐	☐
	13	The student verbalizes that they will document their session in the note.	☐	☐	☐
Other	14 ⚐	The student has optimal body mechanics during performance of the skill.	☐	☐	☐
	15 ⚐	The student uses appropriate therapeutic touch.	☐	☐	☐
	16	The student is able to complete the check-off in the time allotted.	☐	☐	☐
Communication	17	The student uses language the patient can understand.	☐	☐	☐
	18	The student listens actively to the patient during the session.	☐	☐	☐
	19	The student ensures the patient understands instructions by having the patient teach back or demonstrate.	☐	☐	☐
	20 ⚐	The student demonstrates confidence and provides the patient with clear instruction and cueing.	☐	☐	☐

Peer Name (Printed)		**Peer Signature**		**Date of Peer Review**	
Instructor Name (Printed and Signature)	By signing this skills checklist, I am declaring this student competent in the skill described above.			**Date of Instructor Review**	
NOTES					

⚐ = Critical Safety Element/Professionalism. If a student is unable to complete a flagged step without cueing, they will need to return at another time to redo the check-off. All other steps can be cued.

Chapter 9
Developmental Reflexes

Larson T. *Entry-Level Skill Checklists for*
Physical Therapist Assistant Students (pp 105-107).
© 2023 Taylor & Francis Group.

Student Name: _____

Skill		Developmental Reflexes			
Source		Lazaro RT, Umphred DA. *Umphred's Neurorehabilitation for the Physical Therapist Assistant.* 3rd ed. SLACK Incorporated; 2021.	**Check When Completed**		
			Self	Peer	Instructor
Student Introduction and Consent	1 ⌐	The student introduces themself to the patient/caregiver. Must include that they are a **student** PTA and list the school's name.	☐	☐	☐
	2 ⌐	The student verifies the patient's identity. Must use at least 2 patient identifiers (name, date of birth).	☐	☐	☐
	3 ⌐	The student gains consent: • Speaks with the patient/caregiver about their status (acquires relevant information) • Educates the patient/caregiver on intended data collection/intervention and goals for the session • Gains permission to perform said data collection/intervention	☐	☐	☐
Student, Patient, and Supply Preparation	4 ⌐	The student gathers supplies and prepares treatment area (cleans equipment, checks for safety hazards, ensures all equipment is functional and appropriate).	☐	☐	☐
	5	The student washes their hands:			
		Student removes all jewelry from their wrists and hands. Student turns the water to the preferred temperature and wets their hands. Student applies the soap to their hands and washes them with their hands pointed down. Student scrubs for 40–60 seconds and includes palm, between fingers, fingernails, and dorsum of hands. Student rinses hands with hands pointed down. Student dries their hands with a paper towel, uses a paper towel to turn off the water, and then disposes of the paper towel in the trash.	☐	☐	☐
	6	The student places the patient in the correct position for support, comfort, and access to body area necessary for data collection/intervention.	☐	☐	☐
Skill Performance	7	The student correctly assesses **Moro Reflex**:			
		Student holds the infant securely and then drops the infant's head backward and observes the infant's reaction to the motion.	☐	☐	☐
		Student describes expected response if reflex was present: *(Infant will abduct and extend their arms and will most likely cry).*	☐	☐	☐
		Student correctly identifies approximate age of integration: *(3–5 months).*	☐	☐	☐
	8	The student correctly measures **Asymmetrical Tonic Neck Reflex (ATNR)**:			
		Student places the infant in the supine position and rotates their head to one side.	☐	☐	☐
		Student describes expected response if reflex was present: *(Infant will abduct their shoulder and extend their arm on the facial side. On the occipital side, they will flex their elbow and abduct their shoulder).*	☐	☐	☐
		Student correctly identifies approximate age of integration: *(4–5 months).*	☐	☐	☐
	9	The student correctly measures **Symmetrical Tonic Neck Reflex (STNR)**:			
		Student places the infant in the quadruped position and gently moves their neck into extension by holding chin.	☐	☐	☐
		Student describes expected response if reflex was present: *(Infant will flex their knees and extend their arms).*	☐	☐	☐
		Repeat with neck into flexion.	☐	☐	☐
		Student correctly identifies approximate age of integration: *(6–8 months).*	☐	☐	☐

⌐ = Critical Safety Element/Professionalism. If a student is unable to complete a flagged step without cueing, they will need to return at another time to redo the check-off. All other steps can be cued.

	10	The student washes their hands post–skill performance:			
Post-Skill		Student removes all jewelry from their wrists and hands. Student turns the water to the preferred temperature and wets their hands. Student applies the soap to their hands and washes them with their hands pointed down. Student scrubs for 40–60 seconds and includes palm, between fingers, fingernails, and dorsum of hands. Student rinses hands with hands pointed down. Student dries their hands with a paper towel, uses a paper towel to turn off the water, and then disposes of the paper towel in the trash.	☐	☐	☐
	11	The student verbalizes that they will document their session in the note.	☐	☐	☐
Other	12 ⚑	The student has optimal body mechanics during performance of the skill.	☐	☐	☐
	13 ⚑	The student uses appropriate therapeutic touch.	☐	☐	☐
	14	The student is able to complete the check-off in the time allotted.	☐	☐	☐
Communication	15	The student uses language the patient/caregiver can understand.	☐	☐	☐
	16	The student listens actively to the patient/caregiver during the session.	☐	☐	☐
	17	The student ensures the patient/caregiver understands instructions by having the patient/caregiver teach back or demonstrate.	☐	☐	☐
	18 ⚑	The student demonstrates confidence and provides the patient/caregiver with clear instruction and cueing.	☐	☐	☐

Peer Name (Printed)		Peer Signature		Date of Peer Review	
Instructor Name (Printed and Signature)	By signing this skills checklist, I am declaring this student competent in the skill described above.			Date of Instructor Review	
NOTES					

⚑ = Critical Safety Element/Professionalism. If a student is unable to complete a flagged step without cueing, they will need to return at another time to redo the check-off. All other steps can be cued.

Section II

Interventions

Breathing Exercises

Larson T. *Entry-Level Skill Checklists for Physical Therapist Assistant Students* (pp 111-113). © 2023 Taylor & Francis Group.

Student Name: _____

Skill		Breathing Exercises			
Source		Klaczak Kopack J, Cascardi KA. *Principles of Therapeutic Exercise for the Physical Therapist Assistant.* SLACK Incorporated; 2023.	**Check When Completed**		
			Self	Peer	Instructor
Student Introduction and Consent	1 ⚑	The student introduces themself to the patient. Must include that they are a **student** PTA and list the school's name.	☐	☐	☐
	2 ⚑	The student verifies the patient's identity. Must use at least 2 patient identifiers (name, date of birth).	☐	☐	☐
	3 ⚑	The student gains consent: • Speaks with the patient about their status (acquires relevant information) • Educates the patient on intended data collection/intervention and goals for the session • Gains permission to perform said data collection/intervention	☐	☐	☐
Student, Patient, and Supply Preparation	4 ⚑	The student gathers supplies and prepares treatment area (cleans equipment, checks for safety hazards, ensures all equipment is functional and appropriate).	☐	☐	☐
	5	The student washes their hands:			
		Student removes all jewelry from their wrists and hands. Student turns the water to the preferred temperature and wets their hands. Student applies the soap to their hands and washes them with their hands pointed down. Student scrubs for 40–60 seconds and includes palm, between fingers, fingernails, and dorsum of hands. Student rinses hands with hands pointed down. Student dries their hands with a paper towel, uses a paper towel to turn off the water, and then disposes of the paper towel in the trash.	☐	☐	☐
	6	The student places the patient in the correct position for support, comfort, and access to body area necessary for data collection/intervention.	☐	☐	☐
Skill Performance	7	The student correctly instructs the patient in **Diaphragmatic Breathing**:			
		Student correctly explains the purpose of the technique: *(Normalize breathing pattern [decrease accessory muscle use] Help reduce dyspnea Increase ventilation and oxygenation).*	☐	☐	☐
		Student has patient assume a comfortable position (sitting or supine).	☐	☐	☐
		Student instructs patient to place one hand on their stomach and another on their chest.	☐	☐	☐
		Student instructs patient to inhale slowly through their nose (only the hand on their stomach should raise, the hand on the chest should remain still).	☐	☐	☐
		Student instructs patient to exhale slowly through their lips and by actively contracting their abdominals.	☐	☐	☐
		Student educates patient to repeat this for 5–10 minutes, 2–3 times a day.	☐	☐	☐
	8	The student correctly instructs the patient in **Pursed Lip Breathing**:			
		Student correctly explains the purpose of the technique: *(Helps to reduce dyspnea Improves ventilation and oxygenation [relieves respiratory symptoms]).*	☐	☐	☐
		Student has patient sitting in a chair.	☐	☐	☐
		Student instructs patient to breathe in slowly through their nose (mouth closed) for a count of 3–4 seconds and then open the mouth (into a whistling or puckering position) and exhale slowly for a count of 6 seconds.	☐	☐	☐
		Student instructs patient to repeat this anytime they feel short of breath.	☐	☐	☐

⚑ = Critical Safety Element/Professionalism. If a student is unable to complete a flagged step without cueing, they will need to return at another time to redo the check-off. All other steps can be cued.

	9	The student correctly instructs the patient in **Segmental Breathing**:			
		Student correctly explains the purpose of the technique: *(Encourage expansion of segments/areas of the lungs).*	☐	☐	☐
		Student has patient assume a comfortable position (sitting or supine).	☐	☐	☐
		Student places their hands on patient's lateral lower ribs and instructs patient to exhale.	☐	☐	☐
		During exhalation student provides a gentle squeezing pressure and immediately prior to inhalation, provides a quick, gentle stretch down and in (to facilitate contraction of the intercostals).	☐	☐	☐
Post-Skill	10	The student washes their hands post–skill performance:			
		Student removes all jewelry from their wrists and hands. Student turns the water to the preferred temperature and wets their hands. Student applies the soap to their hands and washes them with their hands pointed down. Student scrubs for 40–60 seconds and includes palm, between fingers, fingernails, and dorsum of hands. Student rinses hands with hands pointed down. Student dries their hands with a paper towel, uses a paper towel to turn off the water, and then disposes of the paper towel in the trash.	☐	☐	☐
	11	The student verbalizes that they will document their session in the note.	☐	☐	☐
Other	12 ⚑	The student has optimal body mechanics during performance of the skill.	☐	☐	☐
	13 ⚑	The student uses appropriate therapeutic touch.	☐	☐	☐
	14	The student is able to complete the check-off in the time allotted.	☐	☐	☐
Communication	15	The student uses language the patient can understand.	☐	☐	☐
	16	The student listens actively to the patient during the session.	☐	☐	☐
	17	The student ensures the patient understands instructions by having the patient teach back or demonstrate.	☐	☐	☐
	18 ⚑	The student demonstrates confidence and provides the patient with clear instruction and cueing.	☐	☐	☐

Peer Name (Printed)		Peer Signature		Date of Peer Review	
Instructor Name (Printed and Signature)	By signing this skills checklist, I am declaring this student competent in the skill described above.			Date of Instructor Review	
NOTES					

⚑ = Critical Safety Element/Professionalism. If a student is unable to complete a flagged step without cueing, they will need to return at another time to redo the check-off. All other steps can be cued.

Chapter 11

Airway Clearance

Larson T. *Entry-Level Skill Checklists for Physical Therapist Assistant Students* (pp 115-117).
© 2023 Taylor & Francis Group.

Student Name: _____

Skill		Airway Clearance			
Source		Klaczak Kopack J, Cascardi KA. *Principles of Therapeutic Exercise for the Physical Therapist Assistant.* SLACK Incorporated; 2023.	**Check When Completed**		
			Self	Peer	Instructor
Student Introduction and Consent	1 ⚑	The student introduces themself to the patient. Must include that they are a **student** PTA and list the school's name.	☐	☐	☐
	2 ⚑	The student verifies the patient's identity. Must use at least 2 patient identifiers (name, date of birth).	☐	☐	☐
	3 ⚑	The student gains consent: <ul><li>Speaks with the patient about their status (acquires relevant information)</li><li>Educates the patient on intended data collection/intervention and goals for the session</li><li>Gains permission to perform said data collection/intervention</li></ul>	☐	☐	☐
Student, Patient, and Supply Preparation	4 ⚑	The student gathers supplies and prepares treatment area (cleans equipment, checks for safety hazards, ensures all equipment is functional and appropriate).	☐	☐	☐
	5	The student washes their hands:			
		Student removes all jewelry from their wrists and hands. Student turns the water to the preferred temperature and wets their hands. Student applies the soap to their hands and washes them with their hands pointed down. Student scrubs for 40–60 seconds and includes palm, between fingers, fingernails, and dorsum of hands. Student rinses hands with hands pointed down. Student dries their hands with a paper towel, uses a paper towel to turn off the water, and then disposes of the paper towel in the trash.	☐	☐	☐
	6	The student places the patient in the correct position for support, comfort, and access to body area necessary for data collection/intervention.	☐	☐	☐
Skill Performance	7	The student correctly performs **Postural Drainage and Percussion/Vibration**:			
		Student correctly explains the purpose of postural drainage and percussion/vibration. Student uses language consistent with: *(Both are interventions to help with airway clearance. Postural drainage places the patient in a position to drain a particular lung segment most optimally. Percussion/vibration is a technique to loosen secretions).*	☐	☐	☐
		Student places patient in the correct postural drainage position: *(Left upper lobe: posterior segment: sitting and hugging pillow Left lower lobe: lying on the right side, legs elevated to approximately 18–20 degrees Right lower lobe: lying on the left side, legs elevated to approximately 18–20 degrees).*	☐	☐	☐
		Student explains to patient that these techniques may cause them to cough or spit up sputum. Student provides patient with tissues/towels in which to use for sputum.	☐	☐	☐
		Student performs percussion to correct lobe for 2 minutes: *(Left upper lobe: posterior segment = left upper back region—near the upper trapezius Left lower lobe: left medial trunk—below the scapula Right lower lobe: right medial trunk—below the scapula).*	☐	☐	☐
		Student uses appropriate force, rhythm, and technique during the intervention: *(Moderate force—steady rhythm—hands cupped).*	☐	☐	☐
		Student performs vibration to correct lobe for 5 respirations. Student instructs patient to take a deep breath and provides a vibration force to the chest wall upon exhalation. Repeats for 5 respirations.	☐	☐	☐

⚑ = Critical Safety Element/Professionalism. If a student is unable to complete a flagged step without cueing, they will need to return at another time to redo the check-off. All other steps can be cued.

Post-Skill	8	The student washes their hands post–skill performance:			
		Student removes all jewelry from their wrists and hands. Student turns the water to the preferred temperature and wets their hands. Student applies the soap to their hands and washes them with their hands pointed down. Student scrubs for 40–60 seconds and includes palm, between fingers, fingernails, and dorsum of hands. Student rinses hands with hands pointed down. Student dries their hands with a paper towel, uses a paper towel to turn off the water, and then disposes of the paper towel in the trash.	☐	☐	☐
	9	The student verbalizes that they will document their session in the note.	☐	☐	☐
Other	10 ⚑	The student has optimal body mechanics during performance of the skill.	☐	☐	☐
	11 ⚑	The student uses appropriate therapeutic touch.	☐	☐	☐
	12	The student is able to complete the check-off in the time allotted.	☐	☐	☐
Communication	13	The student uses language the patient can understand.	☐	☐	☐
	14	The student listens actively to the patient during the session.	☐	☐	☐
	15	The student ensures the patient understands instructions by having the patient teach back or demonstrate.	☐	☐	☐
	16 ⚑	The student demonstrates confidence and provides the patient with clear instruction and cueing.	☐	☐	☐

Peer Name (Printed)		Peer Signature		Date of Peer Review	
Instructor Name (Printed and Signature)	By signing this skills checklist, I am declaring this student competent in the skill described above.			Date of Instructor Review	
NOTES					

⚑ = Critical Safety Element/Professionalism. If a student is unable to complete a flagged step without cueing, they will need to return at another time to redo the check-off. All other steps can be cued.

Chapter 12

Physical Agents

Larson T. *Entry-Level Skill Checklists for*
Physical Therapist Assistant Students (pp 119-135).
© 2023 Taylor & Francis Group.

Student Name: _____

Skill		Physical Agents: Electrotherapy—Sensory Level			
Source		Memolo J. *Therapeutic Agents for the Physical Therapist Assistant.* SLACK Incorporated; 2022.	Check When Completed		
			Self	Peer	Instructor
Student Introduction and Consent	1 ⚐	The student introduces themself to the patient. Must include that they are a **student** PTA and list the school's name.	☐	☐	☐
	2 ⚐	The student verifies the patient's identity. Must use at least 2 patient identifiers (name, date of birth).	☐	☐	☐
	3 ⚐	The student gains consent: • Speaks with the patient about their status (acquires relevant information) • Educates the patient on intended data collection/intervention and goals for the session • Gains permission to perform said data collection/intervention	☐	☐	☐
Student, Patient, and Supply Preparation	4 ⚐	The student gathers supplies and prepares treatment area (cleans equipment, checks for safety hazards, ensures all equipment is functional and appropriate).	☐	☐	☐
	5	The student washes their hands:			
		Student removes all jewelry from their wrists and hands. Student turns the water to the preferred temperature and wets their hands. Student applies the soap to their hands and washes them with their hands pointed down. Student scrubs for 40–60 seconds and includes palm, between fingers, fingernails, and dorsum of hands. Student rinses hands with hands pointed down. Student dries their hands with a paper towel, uses a paper towel to turn off the water, and then disposes of the paper towel in the trash.	☐	☐	☐
	6	The student places the patient in the correct position for support, comfort, and access to body area necessary for data collection/intervention.	☐	☐	☐
Skill Performance	7	The student correctly applies **Transcutaneous Electrical Nerve Stimulation (TENS)**:			
		Student assesses the skin and confirms patient does not have any contraindications.	☐	☐	☐
		Student positions patient correctly for the given body part.	☐	☐	☐
		Student places the electrodes to bracket the area of pain.	☐	☐	☐
		Student connects the electrodes to the leads to administer the wavelength desired based on target treatment.	☐	☐	☐
		Student slowly increases the intensity to achieve the desired effect.	☐	☐	☐
		Student provides a way for patient to reach the clinician during treatment as needed.	☐	☐	☐
		Student assesses outcomes after treatment.	☐	☐	☐

⚐ = Critical Safety Element/Professionalism. If a student is unable to complete a flagged step without cueing, they will need to return at another time to redo the check-off. All other steps can be cued.

	8	The student correctly applies **Interferential Current (IFC)**:			
		Student assesses the skin and confirms patient does not have any contraindications.	☐	☐	☐
		Student positions patient correctly for the given body part.	☐	☐	☐
		Student places the electrodes to bracket the area of pain (for larger treatment areas a quadripolar electrode set-up is commonly used).	☐	☐	☐
		Student connects the first set of lead wires in a diagonal and then connects the second set of lead wires to the remaining electrodes in the opposite diagonal.	☐	☐	☐
		Student selects the appropriate treatment parameters to achieve the desired effect and turns on the machine.	☐	☐	☐
		Student slowly increases the intensity to achieve the desired effect.	☐	☐	☐
		Student provides a way for patient to reach the clinician during treatment as needed.	☐	☐	☐
		Student assesses outcomes after treatment.	☐	☐	☐
Post-Skill	9	The student washes their hands post–skill performance:			
		Student removes all jewelry from their wrists and hands. Student turns the water to the preferred temperature and wets their hands. Student applies the soap to their hands and washes them with their hands pointed down. Student scrubs for 40–60 seconds and includes palm, between fingers, fingernails, and dorsum of hands. Student rinses hands with hands pointed down. Student dries their hands with a paper towel, uses a paper towel to turn off the water, and then disposes of the paper towel in the trash.	☐	☐	☐
	10	The student verbalizes that they will document their session in the note.	☐	☐	☐
Other	11 ⚑	The student has optimal body mechanics during performance of the skill.	☐	☐	☐
	12 ⚑	The student uses appropriate therapeutic touch.	☐	☐	☐
	13	The student is able to complete the check-off in the time allotted.	☐	☐	☐
Communication	14	The student uses language the patient can understand.	☐	☐	☐
	15	The student listens actively to the patient during the session.	☐	☐	☐
	16	The student ensures the patient understands instructions by having the patient teach back or demonstrate.	☐	☐	☐
	17 ⚑	The student demonstrates confidence and provides the patient with clear instruction and cueing.	☐	☐	☐

Peer Name (Printed)		**Peer Signature**		**Date of Peer Review**	
Instructor Name (Printed and Signature)	By signing this skills checklist, I am declaring this student competent in the skill described above.			**Date of Instructor Review**	

NOTES	

⚑ = Critical Safety Element/Professionalism. If a student is unable to complete a flagged step without cueing, they will need to return at another time to redo the check-off. All other steps can be cued.

TENS Parameters		
	Conventional High-Rate Sensory TENS	**Low-Rate Motor TENS**
Frequency	100–150 pps	<10 pps
Pulse Duration	50–80 μs	200–300 μs
Amplitude	Sensory	Small muscle contraction
Treatment Time	Unlimited	Maximum 20–30 minutes every 2 hours
Duration of Action	Only while on	4–5 hours after treatment

IFC Parameters				
Purpose	**Frequency**	**Time**	**Modulation**	**Amplitude**
Acute pain	100–150 Hz	Throughout the duration of pain; may be used for 24 hours/day if needed	Use if available	To produce tingling
Chronic pain	2–10 Hz	20–30 minutes	None	To visible contraction

= Critical Safety Element/Professionalism. If a student is unable to complete a flagged step without cueing, they will need to return at another time to redo the check-off. All other steps can be cued.

Student Name: _____

Skill		Physical Agents: Electrotherapy—Motor Level			
Source		Memolo J. *Therapeutic Agents for the Physical Therapist Assistant.* SLACK Incorporated; 2022.	**Check When Completed**		
			Self	Peer	Instructor
Student Introduction and Consent	1 ⚑	The student introduces themself to the patient. Must include that they are a **student** PTA and list the school's name.	☐	☐	☐
	2 ⚑	The student verifies the patient's identity. Must use at least 2 patient identifiers (name, date of birth).	☐	☐	☐
	3 ⚑	The student gains consent: • Speaks with the patient about their status (acquires relevant information) • Educates the patient on intended data collection/intervention and goals for the session • Gains permission to perform said data collection/intervention	☐	☐	☐
Student, Patient, and Supply Preparation	4 ⚑	The student gathers supplies and prepares treatment area (cleans equipment, checks for safety hazards, ensures all equipment is functional and appropriate).	☐	☐	☐
	5	The student washes their hands:			
		Student removes all jewelry from their wrists and hands. Student turns the water to the preferred temperature and wets their hands. Student applies the soap to their hands and washes them with their hands pointed down. Student scrubs for 40–60 seconds and includes palm, between fingers, fingernails, and dorsum of hands. Student rinses hands with hands pointed down. Student dries their hands with a paper towel, uses a paper towel to turn off the water, and then disposes of the paper towel in the trash.	☐	☐	☐
	6	The student places the patient in the correct position for support, comfort, and access to body area necessary for data collection/intervention.	☐	☐	☐
Skill Performance	7	The student correctly applies **Neuromuscular Electrical Stimulation (NMES)**:			
		Student assesses the skin and confirms patient does not have any contraindications.	☐	☐	☐
		Student helps patient into a comfortable position or a functional position depending on the purpose of the NMES treatment.	☐	☐	☐
		Student places one electrode over a muscle belly and the second electrode over the muscle to be stimulated parallel to the muscle fiber direction at least 2 inches away from first electrode.	☐	☐	☐
		Student connects the electrodes to the leads to administer the wavelength desired based on target treatment.	☐	☐	☐
		Student slowly increases the intensity to achieve the desired effect.	☐	☐	☐
		Student instructs patient through functional exercise as indicated.	☐	☐	☐
		Student provides a way for patient to reach the clinician during treatment as needed.	☐	☐	☐
		Student assesses outcomes after treatment.	☐	☐	☐

⚑ = Critical Safety Element/Professionalism. If a student is unable to complete a flagged step without cueing, they will need to return at another time to redo the check-off. All other steps can be cued.

	8	The student washes their hands post–skill performance:			
Post-Skill		Student removes all jewelry from their wrists and hands. Student turns the water to the preferred temperature and wets their hands. Student applies the soap to their hands and washes them with their hands pointed down. Student scrubs for 40–60 seconds and includes palm, between fingers, fingernails, and dorsum of hands. Student rinses hands with hands pointed down. Student dries their hands with a paper towel, uses a paper towel to turn off the water, and then disposes of the paper towel in the trash.	☐	☐	☐
	9	The student verbalizes that they will document their session in the note.	☐	☐	☐
Other	10 ⚑	The student has optimal body mechanics during performance of the skill.	☐	☐	☐
	11 ⚑	The student uses appropriate therapeutic touch.	☐	☐	☐
	12	The student is able to complete the check-off in the time allotted.	☐	☐	☐
Communication	13	The student uses language the patient can understand.	☐	☐	☐
	14	The student listens actively to the patient during the session.	☐	☐	☐
	15	The student ensures the patient understands instructions by having the patient teach back or demonstrate.	☐	☐	☐
	16 ⚑	The student demonstrates confidence and provides the patient with clear instruction and cueing.	☐	☐	☐

Peer Name (Printed)		Peer Signature		Date of Peer Review	
Instructor Name (Printed and Signature)	By signing this skills checklist, I am declaring this student competent in the skill described above.			Date of Instructor Review	
NOTES					

⚑ = Critical Safety Element/Professionalism. If a student is unable to complete a flagged step without cueing, they will need to return at another time to redo the check-off. All other steps can be cued.

NMES Parameters							
Purpose	Pulse Frequency	Pulse Duration	Amplitude	On/Off Time	Ramp Time	Treatment Time	Times Per Day
Muscle Strengthening	35–80 pps	150–200 μs for small muscles

200–350 μs for large muscles | To >10% or MVIC in injured

>50% MVIC in uninjured | 6–10 seconds on, 50–120 seconds off, ratio 1:5 initially | At least 2 seconds | 10–20 minutes to produce 10–20 repetitions | Every 2–3 hours when awake |
| **Muscle Reeducation** | 35–50 pps | 150–200 μs for small muscles

200–350 μs for large muscles | Sufficient for functional activity | Depends on functional activity | At least 2 seconds | Depends on functional activity | N/A |
| **Muscle Spasm Reduction** | 35–50 pps | 150–200 μs for small muscles

200–350 μs for large muscles | To visible contraction | 2–5 seconds on, 2–5 seconds off | At least 1 second | 10–30 minutes | Every 2–3 hours until spasm is relieved |
| **Edema Reduction Using Muscle Pump** | 35–50 pps | 150–200 μs for small muscles

200–350 μs for large muscles | To visible contraction | 2–5 seconds on, 2–5 seconds off | At least 1 second | 30 minutes | Twice a day |

⌐⌐ = Critical Safety Element/Professionalism. If a student is unable to complete a flagged step without cueing, they will need to return at another time to redo the check-off. All other steps can be cued.

Student Name: _____

Skill		Physical Agents: Cryotherapy			
Source		Memolo J. *Therapeutic Agents for the Physical Therapist Assistant.* SLACK Incorporated; 2022.	**Check When Completed**		
			Self	Peer	Instructor
Student Introduction and Consent	1 ⚑	The student introduces themself to the patient. Must include that they are a **student** PTA and list the school's name.	☐	☐	☐
	2 ⚑	The student verifies the patient's identity. Must use at least 2 patient identifiers (name, date of birth).	☐	☐	☐
	3 ⚑	The student gains consent: • Speaks with the patient about their status (acquires relevant information) • Educates the patient on intended data collection/intervention and goals for the session • Gains permission to perform said data collection/intervention	☐	☐	☐
Student, Patient, and Supply Preparation	4 ⚑	The student gathers supplies and prepares treatment area (cleans equipment, checks for safety hazards, ensures all equipment is functional and appropriate).	☐	☐	☐
	5	The student washes their hands:			
		Student removes all jewelry from their wrists and hands. Student turns the water to the preferred temperature and wets their hands. Student applies the soap to their hands and washes them with their hands pointed down. Student scrubs for 40–60 seconds and includes palm, between fingers, fingernails, and dorsum of hands. Student rinses hands with hands pointed down. Student dries their hands with a paper towel, uses a paper towel to turn off the water, and then disposes of the paper towel in the trash.	☐	☐	☐
	6	The student places the patient in the correct position for support, comfort, and access to body area necessary for data collection/intervention.	☐	☐	☐
Skill Performance	7	The student correctly applies **Cold Pack**:			
		Student assesses the skin and confirms patient does not have any contraindications.	☐	☐	☐
		Student positions patient correctly for the given body part.	☐	☐	☐
		Student applies the cold pack to the skin and covers it with a towel. Student secures it in place with elastic strap or plastic wrap.	☐	☐	☐
		Student applies the cold pack and provides patient with a call bell.	☐	☐	☐
		After 5 minutes, student checks patient's skin.	☐	☐	☐
		Total treatment time: 10–20 minutes.	☐	☐	☐
		Once treatment is completed, student assesses patient's skin.	☐	☐	☐
	8	The student correctly applies **Ice Massage**:			
		Student assesses the skin and confirms patient does not have any contraindications.	☐	☐	☐
		Student positions patient correctly for the given body part.	☐	☐	☐
		Student applies the ice directly to the skin and on the location of pain in small circles.	☐	☐	☐
		Ice massage should be continued until patient receives analgesia. Total treatment time is less than cold pack.	☐	☐	☐
		Once treatment is completed, student assesses patient's skin.	☐	☐	☐

⚑ = Critical Safety Element/Professionalism. If a student is unable to complete a flagged step without cueing, they will need to return at another time to redo the check-off. All other steps can be cued.

	9	The student washes their hands post–skill performance:			
Post-Skill		Student removes all jewelry from their wrists and hands. Student turns the water to the preferred temperature and wets their hands. Student applies the soap to their hands and washes them with their hands pointed down. Student scrubs for 40–60 seconds and includes palm, between fingers, fingernails, and dorsum of hands. Student rinses hands with hands pointed down. Student dries their hands with a paper towel, uses a paper towel to turn off the water, and then disposes of the paper towel in the trash.	☐	☐	☐
	10	The student verbalizes that they will document their session in the note.	☐	☐	☐
Other	11 ⚑	The student has optimal body mechanics during performance of the skill.	☐	☐	☐
	12 ⚑	The student uses appropriate therapeutic touch.	☐	☐	☐
	13	The student is able to complete the check-off in the time allotted.	☐	☐	☐
Communication	14	The student uses language the patient can understand.	☐	☐	☐
	15	The student listens actively to the patient during the session.	☐	☐	☐
	16	The student ensures the patient understands instructions by having the patient teach back or demonstrate.	☐	☐	☐
	17 ⚑	The student demonstrates confidence and provides the patient with clear instruction and cueing.	☐	☐	☐

Peer Name (Printed)		**Peer Signature**		**Date of Peer Review**	
Instructor Name (Printed and Signature)	By signing this skills checklist, I am declaring this student competent in the skill described above.			**Date of Instructor Review**	
NOTES					

⚑ = Critical Safety Element/Professionalism. If a student is unable to complete a flagged step without cueing, they will need to return at another time to redo the check-off. All other steps can be cued.

Student Name: _____

Skill		Physical Agents: Moist Hot Pack			
Source		Memolo J. *Therapeutic Agents for the Physical Therapist Assistant.* SLACK Incorporated; 2022.	**Check When Completed**		
			Self	Peer	Instructor
Student Introduction and Consent	1 ⚑	The student introduces themself to the patient. Must include that they are a **student** PTA and list the school's name.	☐	☐	☐
	2 ⚑	The student verifies the patient's identity. Must use at least 2 patient identifiers (name, date of birth).	☐	☐	☐
	3 ⚑	The student gains consent: • Speaks with the patient about their status (acquires relevant information) • Educates the patient on intended data collection/intervention and goals for the session • Gains permission to perform said data collection/intervention	☐	☐	☐
Student, Patient, and Supply Preparation	4 ⚑	The student gathers supplies and prepares treatment area (cleans equipment, checks for safety hazards, ensures all equipment is functional and appropriate).	☐	☐	☐
	5	The student washes their hands:			
		Student removes all jewelry from their wrists and hands. Student turns the water to the preferred temperature and wets their hands. Student applies the soap to their hands and washes them with their hands pointed down. Student scrubs for 40–60 seconds and includes palm, between fingers, fingernails, and dorsum of hands. Student rinses hands with hands pointed down. Student dries their hands with a paper towel, uses a paper towel to turn off the water, and then disposes of the paper towel in the trash.	☐	☐	☐
	6	The student places the patient in the correct position for support, comfort, and access to body area necessary for data collection/intervention.	☐	☐	☐
Skill Performance	7	The student correctly applies **Moist Hot Pack**:			
	⚑	Student assesses the skin and confirms patient does not have any contraindications.	☐	☐	☐
		Student positions patient correctly for the given body part. **Avoid positioning patient so they are lying on the hot pack.**	☐	☐	☐
		Student prepares the hot pack and correct number of towel layers: *(Traditional moist hot packs = 6–8 layers Gel-filled moist hot packs = 1–3 layers).*	☐	☐	☐
		Student applies the hot pack and provides patient with a call bell.	☐	☐	☐
		After 5 minutes, student checks patient's skin to ensure the correct number of layers.	☐	☐	☐
		Total treatment time can be up to 30 minutes.	☐	☐	☐
		Once treatment is completed, student assesses patient's skin.	☐	☐	☐

⚑ = Critical Safety Element/Professionalism. If a student is unable to complete a flagged step without cueing, they will need to return at another time to redo the check-off. All other steps can be cued.

	8	The student washes their hands post–skill performance:			
Post-Skill		Student removes all jewelry from their wrists and hands. Student turns the water to the preferred temperature and wets their hands. Student applies the soap to their hands and washes them with their hands pointed down. Student scrubs for 40–60 seconds and includes palm, between fingers, fingernails, and dorsum of hands. Student rinses hands with hands pointed down. Student dries their hands with a paper towel, uses a paper towel to turn off the water, and then disposes of the paper towel in the trash.	☐	☐	☐
	9	The student verbalizes that they will document their session in the note.	☐	☐	☐
Other	10 ⚑	The student has optimal body mechanics during performance of the skill.	☐	☐	☐
	11 ⚑	The student uses appropriate therapeutic touch.	☐	☐	☐
	12	The student is able to complete the check-off in the time allotted.	☐	☐	☐
Communication	13	The student uses language the patient can understand.	☐	☐	☐
	14	The student listens actively to the patient during the session.	☐	☐	☐
	15	The student ensures the patient understands instructions by having the patient teach back or demonstrate.	☐	☐	☐
	16 ⚑	The student demonstrates confidence and provides the patient with clear instruction and cueing.	☐	☐	☐
Peer Name (Printed)			**Peer Signature**		**Date of Peer Review**	
Instructor Name (Printed and Signature)	By signing this skills checklist, I am declaring this student competent in the skill described above.				**Date of Instructor Review**	
NOTES						

⚑ = Critical Safety Element/Professionalism. If a student is unable to complete a flagged step without cueing, they will need to return at another time to redo the check-off. All other steps can be cued.

Student Name: _____

Skill		Physical Agents: Paraffin			
Source		Memolo J. *Therapeutic Agents for the Physical Therapist Assistant.* SLACK Incorporated; 2022.	Check When Completed		
			Self	Peer	Instructor
Student Introduction and Consent	1 ⚑	The student introduces themself to the patient. Must include that they are a **student** PTA and list the school's name.	☐	☐	☐
	2 ⚑	The student verifies the patient's identity. Must use at least 2 patient identifiers (name, date of birth).	☐	☐	☐
	3 ⚑	The student gains consent: • Speaks with the patient about their status (acquires relevant information) • Educates the patient on intended data collection/intervention and goals for the session • Gains permission to perform said data collection/intervention	☐	☐	☐
Student, Patient, and Supply Preparation	4 ⚑	The student gathers supplies and prepares treatment area (cleans equipment, checks for safety hazards, ensures all equipment is functional and appropriate).	☐	☐	☐
	5	The student washes their hands:			
		Student removes all jewelry from their wrists and hands. Student turns the water to the preferred temperature and wets their hands. Student applies the soap to their hands and washes them with their hands pointed down. Student scrubs for 40–60 seconds and includes palm, between fingers, fingernails, and dorsum of hands. Student rinses hands with hands pointed down. Student dries their hands with a paper towel, uses a paper towel to turn off the water, and then disposes of the paper towel in the trash.	☐	☐	☐
	6	The student places the patient in the correct position for support, comfort, and access to body area necessary for data collection/intervention.	☐	☐	☐
Skill Performance	7	The student correctly applies **Paraffin**:			
		Student ensures all jewelry is removed and inspects the skin for open wounds, infections, or new scar tissue. Student also confirms patient does not have any contraindications.	☐	☐	☐
		Student washes and dries the treatment area.	☐	☐	☐
		Dip-wrap method: Student instructs patient to dip the body part into the wax and bring it back out. Student waits until the wax solidifies and then dips again. This process repeats 6–10 times. After the last dip, the body part is wrapped in plastic wrap and then a towel for 15 minutes.	☐	☐	☐
		Dip-immersion method: Student instructs patient to dip the body part into the wax and bring it back out. Student waits until the wax solidifies and then dips again. Patient keeps the body part in the unplugged tub for the duration of the treatment (up to 20 minutes).	☐	☐	☐
		Paint method: Student paints the wax onto patient using a paint brush. Student waits until the wax solidifies between each painted layer for a total of 6–10 layers. After the last layer, the body part is wrapped in plastic wrap and then a towel for 10–20 minutes.	☐	☐	☐
		After application of paraffin, student removes the wax, inspects the skin, and disposes of the used wax.	☐	☐	☐

⚑ = Critical Safety Element/Professionalism. If a student is unable to complete a flagged step without cueing, they will need to return at another time to redo the check-off. All other steps can be cued.

Post-Skill	8	The student washes their hands post–skill performance:			
		Student removes all jewelry from their wrists and hands. Student turns the water to the preferred temperature and wets their hands. Student applies the soap to their hands and washes them with their hands pointed down. Student scrubs for 40–60 seconds and includes palm, between fingers, fingernails, and dorsum of hands. Student rinses hands with hands pointed down. Student dries their hands with a paper towel, uses a paper towel to turn off the water, and then disposes of the paper towel in the trash.	☐	☐	☐
	9	The student verbalizes that they will document their session in the note.	☐	☐	☐
Other	10 ⚑	The student has optimal body mechanics during performance of the skill.	☐	☐	☐
	11 ⚑	The student uses appropriate therapeutic touch.	☐	☐	☐
	12	The student is able to complete the check-off in the time allotted.	☐	☐	☐
Communication	13	The student uses language the patient can understand.	☐	☐	☐
	14	The student listens actively to the patient during the session.	☐	☐	☐
	15	The student ensures the patient understands instructions by having the patient teach back or demonstrate.	☐	☐	☐
	16 ⚑	The student demonstrates confidence and provides the patient with clear instruction and cueing.	☐	☐	☐

Peer Name (Printed)		**Peer Signature**		**Date of Peer Review**	
Instructor Name (Printed and Signature)	By signing this skills checklist, I am declaring this student competent in the skill described above.			**Date of Instructor Review**	
NOTES					

⚑ = Critical Safety Element/Professionalism. If a student is unable to complete a flagged step without cueing, they will need to return at another time to redo the check-off. All other steps can be cued.

Student Name: _____

Skill		Physical Agents: Ultrasound			
Source		Memolo J. *Therapeutic Agents for the Physical Therapist Assistant.* SLACK Incorporated; 2022.	**Check When Completed**		
			Self	Peer	Instructor
Student Introduction and Consent	1 ⚐	The student introduces themself to the patient. Must include that they are a **student** PTA and list the school's name.	☐	☐	☐
	2 ⚐	The student verifies the patient's identity. Must use at least 2 patient identifiers (name, date of birth).	☐	☐	☐
	3 ⚐	The student gains consent: • Speaks with the patient about their status (acquires relevant information) • Educates the patient on intended data collection/intervention and goals for the session • Gains permission to perform said data collection/intervention	☐	☐	☐
Student, Patient, and Supply Preparation	4 ⚐	The student gathers supplies and prepares treatment area (cleans equipment, checks for safety hazards, ensures all equipment is functional and appropriate).	☐	☐	☐
	5	The student washes their hands:			
		Student removes all jewelry from their wrists and hands. Student turns the water to the preferred temperature and wets their hands. Student applies the soap to their hands and washes them with their hands pointed down. Student scrubs for 40–60 seconds and includes palm, between fingers, fingernails, and dorsum of hands. Student rinses hands with hands pointed down. Student dries their hands with a paper towel, uses a paper towel to turn off the water, and then disposes of the paper towel in the trash.	☐	☐	☐
	6	The student places the patient in the correct position for support, comfort, and access to body area necessary for data collection/intervention.	☐	☐	☐
Skill Performance	7	The student correctly applies **Ultrasound**:			
		Student assesses the skin and confirms patient does not have any contraindications.	☐	☐	☐
		Student positions patient correctly for the given body part.	☐	☐	☐
		Student selects the correct duty cycle based on their goal of treatment: *(Continuous = pain relief, tissue stretch* *Pulsed = tissue healing, inflammatory response).*	☐	☐	☐
		Student selects the correct frequency based on their goal of treatment: *(3 MHz = < 2.5 cm depth* *1 MHz = 2.5–5 cm depth).*	☐	☐	☐
		Student selects the correct intensity based on their goal of treatment: *(Acute injuries = 0.1–0.3 W/cm²* *Subacute injuries = 0.2–0.5 W/cm²* *Chronic injuries = 0.03–0.8 W/cm²).*	☐	☐	☐
		Student selects the correct treatment time based on their goal of treatment: *(2 times the effective radiation area).*	☐	☐	☐
		Student correctly applies a coupling medium.	☐	☐	☐
		Student performs the ultrasound treatment being sure to move the sound head in slow movements over the entire area.	☐	☐	☐
		Once treatment is completed, student cleans and assesses patient's skin.			

⚐ = Critical Safety Element/Professionalism. If a student is unable to complete a flagged step without cueing, they will need to return at another time to redo the check-off. All other steps can be cued.

Post-Skill	8	The student washes their hands post–skill performance:			
		Student removes all jewelry from their wrists and hands. Student turns the water to the preferred temperature and wets their hands. Student applies the soap to their hands and washes them with their hands pointed down. Student scrubs for 40–60 seconds and includes palm, between fingers, fingernails, and dorsum of hands. Student rinses hands with hands pointed down. Student dries their hands with a paper towel, uses a paper towel to turn off the water, and then disposes of the paper towel in the trash.	☐	☐	☐
	9	The student verbalizes that they will document their session in the note.	☐	☐	☐
Other	10 ⚑	The student has optimal body mechanics during performance of the skill.	☐	☐	☐
	11 ⚑	The student uses appropriate therapeutic touch.	☐	☐	☐
	12	The student is able to complete the check-off in the time allotted.	☐	☐	☐
Communication	13	The student uses language the patient can understand.	☐	☐	☐
	14	The student listens actively to the patient during the session.	☐	☐	☐
	15	The student ensures the patient understands instructions by having the patient teach back or demonstrate.	☐	☐	☐
	16 ⚑	The student demonstrates confidence and provides the patient with clear instruction and cueing.	☐	☐	☐

Peer Name (Printed)		**Peer Signature**		**Date of Peer Review**	
Instructor Name (Printed and Signature)	By signing this skills checklist, I am declaring this student competent in the skill described above.			**Date of Instructor Review**	
NOTES					

⚑ = Critical Safety Element/Professionalism. If a student is unable to complete a flagged step without cueing, they will need to return at another time to redo the check-off. All other steps can be cued.

Student Name: _____

Skill		Physical Agents: Mechanical Traction			
Source		Memolo J. *Therapeutic Agents for the Physical Therapist Assistant.* SLACK Incorporated; 2022.	**Check When Completed**		
			Self	Peer	Instructor
Student Introduction and Consent	1 ⚐	The student introduces themself to the patient. Must include that they are a **student** PTA and list the school's name.	☐	☐	☐
	2 ⚐	The student verifies the patient's identity. Must use at least 2 patient identifiers (name, date of birth).	☐	☐	☐
	3 ⚐	The student gains consent: • Speaks with the patient about their status (acquires relevant information) • Educates the patient on intended data collection/intervention and goals for the session • Gains permission to perform said data collection/intervention	☐	☐	☐
Student, Patient, and Supply Preparation	4 ⚐	The student gathers supplies and prepares treatment area (cleans equipment, checks for safety hazards, ensures all equipment is functional and appropriate).	☐	☐	☐
	5	The student washes their hands:			
		Student removes all jewelry from their wrists and hands. Student turns the water to the preferred temperature and wets their hands. Student applies the soap to their hands and washes them with their hands pointed down. Student scrubs for 40–60 seconds and includes palm, between fingers, fingernails, and dorsum of hands. Student rinses hands with hands pointed down. Student dries their hands with a paper towel, uses a paper towel to turn off the water, and then disposes of the paper towel in the trash.	☐	☐	☐
	6	The student places the patient in the correct position for support, comfort, and access to body area necessary for data collection/intervention.	☐	☐	☐
Skill Performance	7	The student correctly applies **Cervical Traction**:			
		Student determines that patient does not have any contraindications.	☐	☐	☐
		Student positions patient in supine on the traction table with their hips and knees flexed at 90 degrees over a stool or bolster.	☐	☐	☐
		Student adjusts the angle of cervical flexion based on their goal of treatment: *(0–5 degrees = upper cervical spine* *10–20 degrees = mid cervical spine* *25–35 degrees = lower cervical spine).*	☐	☐	☐
		Student aligns and secures the straps correctly to the traction table. Student ensures that the straps are tight enough to prevent sliding.	☐	☐	☐
		Student selects the correct force of pull based on their goal of treatment: *(11–15 pounds = tissue stretch/muscle spasms* *20–30 pounds = vertebrae distraction).*	☐	☐	☐
		Student selects the correct type of pull (sustained or intermittent) based on their goal of treatment.	☐	☐	☐
		Student selects the correct on/off times if intermittent: *(Hold time = 15–60 seconds* *Relax time = 5–20 seconds).*	☐	☐	☐
		Student selects the correct treatment duration: *(8–15 minutes).*	☐	☐	☐
		Student provides patient with the emergency stop button and call bell.			

⚐ = Critical Safety Element/Professionalism. If a student is unable to complete a flagged step without cueing, they will need to return at another time to redo the check-off. All other steps can be cued.

	8	The student correctly applies **Lumbar Traction**:			
		Student determines that patient does not have any contraindications.	☐	☐	☐
		Student correctly applies the belts and straps and then assists patient as needed onto the table.	☐	☐	☐
		Student positions patient in supine on the traction table with their hips and knees flexed at 90 degrees over a stool or bolster.	☐	☐	☐
		Student aligns and secures the belts correctly to the traction table. Ensure that the belts are tight enough to prevent sliding.	☐	☐	☐
		Student selects the correct force of pull based on their goal of treatment: *(65–70 pounds or <50% of body weight).*	☐	☐	☐
		Student selects the correct type of pull (sustained or intermittent) based on their goal of treatment.	☐	☐	☐
		Student selects the correct on/off times if intermittent: *(Hold time = 15–60 seconds Relax time = 5–20 seconds).*	☐	☐	☐
		Student selects the correct treatment duration: *(8–15 minutes).*	☐	☐	☐
		Student provides patient with the emergency stop button and call bell.	☐	☐	☐
Post-Skill	9	The student washes their hands post–skill performance:			
		Student removes all jewelry from their wrists and hands. Student turns the water to the preferred temperature and wets their hands. Student applies the soap to their hands and washes them with their hands pointed down. Student scrubs for 40–60 seconds and includes palm, between fingers, fingernails, and dorsum of hands. Student rinses hands with hands pointed down. Student dries their hands with a paper towel, uses a paper towel to turn off the water, and then disposes of the paper towel in the trash.	☐	☐	☐
	10	The student verbalizes that they will document their session in the note.	☐	☐	☐
Other	11 ⚑	The student has optimal body mechanics during performance of the skill.	☐	☐	☐
	12 ⚑	The student uses appropriate therapeutic touch.	☐	☐	☐
	13	The student is able to complete the check-off in the time allotted.	☐	☐	☐
Communication	14	The student uses language the patient can understand.	☐	☐	☐
	15	The student listens actively to the patient during the session.	☐	☐	☐
	16	The student ensures the patient understands instructions by having the patient teach back or demonstrate.	☐	☐	☐
	17 ⚑	The student demonstrates confidence and provides the patient with clear instruction and cueing.	☐	☐	☐

Peer Name (Printed)		**Peer Signature**		**Date of Peer Review**	
Instructor Name (Printed and Signature)	By signing this skills checklist, I am declaring this student competent in the skill described above.			**Date of Instructor Review**	

NOTES	

⚑ = Critical Safety Element/Professionalism. If a student is unable to complete a flagged step without cueing, they will need to return at another time to redo the check-off. All other steps can be cued.

Chapter 13

Functional Training

Larson T. *Entry-Level Skill Checklists for Physical Therapist Assistant Students* (pp 137-160).
© 2023 Taylor & Francis Group.

Student Name: _____

Skill		Functional Training: Positioning and Draping			
Source		Memolo J. *Procedures and Patient Care for the Physical Therapist Assistant.* SLACK Incorporated; 2019.	Check When Completed		
			Self	Peer	Instructor
Student Introduction and Consent	1 ⚐	The student introduces themself to the patient. Must include that they are a **student** PTA and list the school's name.	☐	☐	☐
	2 ⚐	The student verifies the patient's identity. Must use at least 2 patient identifiers (name, date of birth).	☐	☐	☐
	3 ⚐	The student gains consent: • Speaks with the patient about their status (acquires relevant information) • Educates the patient on intended data collection/intervention and goals for the session • Gains permission to perform said data collection/intervention	☐	☐	☐
Student, Patient, and Supply Preparation	4 ⚐	The student gathers supplies and prepares treatment area (cleans equipment, checks for safety hazards, ensures all equipment is functional and appropriate).	☐	☐	☐
	5	The student washes their hands:			
		Student removes all jewelry from their wrists and hands. Student turns the water to the preferred temperature and wets their hands. Student applies the soap to their hands and washes them with their hands pointed down. Student scrubs for 40–60 seconds and includes palm, between fingers, fingernails, and dorsum of hands. Student rinses hands with hands pointed down. Student dries their hands with a paper towel, uses a paper towel to turn off the water, and then disposes of the paper towel in the trash.	☐	☐	☐
	6	The student positions patient in the correct position for support, comfort, and access to body area necessary for data collection/intervention.	☐	☐	☐
	7	The student educates the patient on the importance of proper positioning: *(Prevents injury, pressure, and contractures / Provides patient comfort / Provides trunk support and stability / Provides access to areas to be treated / Promotes efficient function of body systems).*	☐	☐	☐
	8	The student educates the patient on the importance of proper draping: *(Provides modesty for patient / Provides warmth for patient / Allows access to areas being treated / Protects clothing from being soiled).*	☐	☐	☐
Skill Performance	9	The student correctly positions the patient in **Supine**:			
		Student lists for the instructor the common bony landmarks at risk in this position: *(Occipital tuberosity, scapulae, posterior iliac spines, spinous processes, sacrum, ischium, medial epicondyle of the humerus, posterior calcanei).*	☐	☐	☐
		Student places a small pillow under the head of patient; avoid excessive neck flexion.	☐	☐	☐
		Student places a thin pillow under patient's knees to decrease pressure on low back; avoid excessive knee flexion.	☐	☐	☐
		Student places a towel roll just proximal to the calcaneus to float the heels.	☐	☐	☐
		Student demonstrates proper draping for upper and lower extremity passive range of motion in this position.	☐	☐	☐

⚐ = Critical Safety Element/Professionalism. If a student is unable to complete a flagged step without cueing, they will need to return at another time to redo the check-off. All other steps can be cued.

	10	The student correctly positions the patient in **Prone**:			
		Student lists for the instructor the bony landmarks at risk in this position: *(Forehead, lateral ear, anterior acromion process, ASIS, anterior head of humerus, dorsum of foot, patella).*	☐	☐	☐
		Student places a small pillow (or towel roll) under patient's forehead; avoid excessive neck extension.	☐	☐	☐
		Student places a pillow under patient's abdomen or anterior lower legs to decrease pressure on the low back.	☐	☐	☐
		Student instructs patient to place their arms in a T position or down by their sides (patient preference).	☐	☐	☐
		Student demonstrates proper draping for low back manual therapy in this position.	☐	☐	☐
	11	The student correctly positions the patient in **Sidelying**:			
		Student lists for the instructor the bony landmarks at risk in this position: *(Lateral ear, lateral ribs, lateral acromion process, lateral head of humerus, medial/lateral epicondyle of the humerus, greater trochanter of femur, medial/lateral condyles of femur, medial/lateral malleoli, 5th metatarsal of foot).*	☐	☐	☐
		Student places a thin pillow under the head of patient.	☐	☐	☐
		Student ensures patient is not positioned directly on their shoulders (patient should be rotated slightly forward or backward to prevent direct pressure on the acromion).	☐	☐	☐
		Student flexes patient's lower extremities (often, the upper leg is slightly more flexed) and places a pillow between patient's knees.	☐	☐	☐
		Student places a pillow across patient's chest and their arms wrapped around it (patient preference).	☐	☐	☐
		Student demonstrates proper draping for exposing the lateral hip in this position.	☐	☐	☐
	12	The student correctly positions the patient in **Sitting**:			
		Student lists for the instructor the bony landmarks at risk in this position: *(Ischial tuberosities, scapular and vertebral processes, sacrum, medial epicondyle of humerus, calcanei).*	☐	☐	☐
		Student ensures that patient's feet can touch the floor and the back is supported in a midline position.	☐	☐	☐
		Student ensures there is no pressure on the popliteal space and the upper extremity support is appropriate.	☐	☐	☐
		Student demonstrates proper draping for exposing the posterior shoulder/scapula in this position.	☐	☐	☐
Post-Skill	13	The student washes their hands post–skill performance:			
		Student removes all jewelry from their wrists and hands. Student turns the water to the preferred temperature and wets their hands. Student applies the soap to their hands and washes them with their hands pointed down. Student scrubs for 40–60 seconds and includes palm, between fingers, fingernails, and dorsum of hands. Student rinses hands with hands pointed down. Student dries their hands with a paper towel, uses a paper towel to turn off the water, and then disposes of the paper towel in the trash.	☐	☐	☐
	14	The student verbalizes that they will document their session in the note.	☐	☐	☐

☐ = Critical Safety Element/Professionalism. If a student is unable to complete a flagged step without cueing, they will need to return at another time to redo the check-off. All other steps can be cued.

Other	15 ⚐	The student has optimal body mechanics during performance of the skill.		☐	☐		☐
	16 ⚐	The student uses appropriate therapeutic touch.		☐	☐		☐
	17	The student is able to complete the check-off in the time allotted.		☐	☐		☐
Communication	18	The student uses language the patient can understand.		☐	☐		☐
	19	The student listens actively to the patient during the session.		☐	☐		☐
	20	The student ensures the patient understands instructions by having the patient teach back or demonstrate.		☐	☐		☐
	21 ⚐	The student demonstrates confidence and provides the patient with clear instruction and cueing.		☐	☐		☐
Peer Name (Printed)			**Peer Signature**			**Date of Peer Review**	
Instructor Name (Printed and Signature)	By signing this skills checklist, I am declaring this student competent in the skill described above.					**Date of Instructor Review**	
NOTES							

⚐ = Critical Safety Element/Professionalism. If a student is unable to complete a flagged step without cueing, they will need to return at another time to redo the check-off. All other steps can be cued.

Student Name: _____

Skill		Functional Training: Bed Mobility			
Source		Memolo J. *Procedures and Patient Care for the Physical Therapist Assistant.* SLACK Incorporated; 2019.	**Check When Completed**		
			Self	Peer	Instructor
Student Introduction and Consent	1 ⚑	The student introduces themself to the patient. Must include that they are a **student** PTA and list the school's name.	☐	☐	☐
	2 ⚑	The student verifies the patient's identity. Must use at least 2 patient identifiers (name, date of birth).	☐	☐	☐
	3 ⚑	The student gains consent: • Speaks with the patient about their status (acquires relevant information) • Educates the patient on intended data collection/intervention and goals for the session • Gains permission to perform said data collection/intervention	☐	☐	☐
Student, Patient, and Supply Preparation	4 ⚑	The student gathers supplies and prepares treatment area (cleans equipment, checks for safety hazards, ensures all equipment is functional and appropriate).	☐	☐	☐
	5	The student washes their hands:			
		Student removes all jewelry from their wrists and hands. Student turns the water to the preferred temperature and wets their hands. Student applies the soap to their hands and washes them with their hands pointed down. Student scrubs for 40–60 seconds and includes palm, between fingers, fingernails, and dorsum of hands. Student rinses hands with hands pointed down. Student dries their hands with a paper towel, uses a paper towel to turn off the water, and then disposes of the paper towel in the trash.	☐	☐	☐
	6	The student places the patient in the correct position for support, comfort, and access to body area necessary for data collection/intervention	☐	☐	☐
Skill Performance	7	The student correctly performs **Rolling**:			
		Student positions patient to the side of the bed opposite the direction they will roll.	☐	☐	☐
		For dependent patients, student crosses their ankles (the top leg opposite of the direction they are rolling).	☐	☐	☐
		For patients who can help, the student asks them to bend the knee on the leg opposite of the direction they will roll. Patient can then use this leg to push into the bed to assist with the roll.	☐	☐	☐
	8	The student correctly performs **Scooting Up/Down**:			
		Student lowers the head of the bed so it is flat and removes pillows/blankets so the movement can be unrestricted.	☐	☐	☐
		For dependent patients, student can place a folded sheet under patient to assist with mobility. One clinician stands on either side of patient and grasps the draw sheet and at the same time pull patient up/down in bed.	☐	☐	☐
		For patients who can help, student instructs them to perform a bridge. To move up in bed, patient will press down with their elbows to assist with lifting the buttocks and back and then pushes with their lower extremities.	☐	☐	☐
		To move down, student instructs patient to bridge and use their elbows to lift, except this time patient will lift and move down in bed.	☐	☐	☐

⚑ = Critical Safety Element/Professionalism. If a student is unable to complete a flagged step without cueing, they will need to return at another time to redo the check-off. All other steps can be cued.

	9	The student correctly performs **Supine to Sit**:			
	⚑	*For dependent patients*, student crosses their ankles (the top leg opposite of the direction they are rolling). Student rolls patient to their side and uses their body to block patient from rolling off the bed.	☐	☐	☐
		While staying close to patient, student uses one arm to hook behind patient's knees while the other arm comes under patient's shoulders. **Do not pull on patient's arms or leg to perform this task.**	☐	☐	☐
	⚑	Student lowers patient's legs down while lifting the shoulders and trunk up. At this point, patient should be sitting on the edge of the bed. **Do not leave patient alone while sitting on edge of bed.**	☐	☐	☐
		For patients who can help, student cues them to roll or scoot to the edge of the bed. Patient should be in sidelying near the edge.	☐	☐	☐
		Student instructs patient to lower their lower extremities to the floor while using their upper extremities to push upright while providing the necessary assistance.	☐	☐	☐
Post-Skill	10	The student washes their hands post–skill performance:			
		Student removes all jewelry from their wrists and hands. Student turns the water to the preferred temperature and wets their hands. Student applies the soap to their hands and washes them with their hands pointed down. Student scrubs for 40–60 seconds and includes palm, between fingers, fingernails, and dorsum of hands. Student rinses hands with hands pointed down. Student dries their hands with a paper towel, uses a paper towel to turn off the water, and then disposes of the paper towel in the trash.	☐	☐	☐
	11	The student verbalizes that they will document their session in the note.	☐	☐	☐
Other	12 ⚑	The student has optimal body mechanics during performance of the skill.	☐	☐	☐
	13 ⚑	The student uses appropriate therapeutic touch.	☐	☐	☐
	14	The student is able to complete the check-off in the time allotted.	☐	☐	☐
Communication	15	The student uses language the patient can understand.	☐	☐	☐
	16	The student listens actively to the patient during the session.	☐	☐	☐
	17	The student ensures the patient understands instructions by having the patient teach back or demonstrate.	☐	☐	☐
	18 ⚑	The student demonstrates confidence and provides the patient with clear instruction and cueing.	☐	☐	☐

Peer Name (Printed)		**Peer Signature**		**Date of Peer Review**	
Instructor Name (Printed and Signature)	By signing this skills checklist, I am declaring this student competent in the skill described above.			**Date of Instructor Review**	
NOTES					

⚑ = Critical Safety Element/Professionalism. If a student is unable to complete a flagged step without cueing, they will need to return at another time to redo the check-off. All other steps can be cued.

Student Name: _____

Skill		Functional Training: Transfers			
Source		Memolo J. *Procedures and Patient Care for the Physical Therapist Assistant.* SLACK Incorporated; 2019.	**Check When Completed**		
			Self	Peer	Instructor
Student Introduction and Consent	1 ⚐	The student introduces themself to the patient. Must include that they are a **student** PTA and list the school's name.	☐	☐	☐
	2 ⚐	The student verifies the patient's identity. Must use at least 2 patient identifiers (name, date of birth).	☐	☐	☐
	3 ⚐	The student gains consent: • Speaks with the patient about their status (acquires relevant information) • Educates the patient on intended data collection/intervention and goals for the session • Gains permission to perform said data collection/intervention	☐	☐	☐
Student, Patient, and Supply Preparation	4 ⚐	The student gathers supplies and prepares treatment area (cleans equipment, checks for safety hazards, ensures all equipment is functional and appropriate).	☐	☐	☐
	5	The student washes their hands:			
		Student removes all jewelry from their wrists and hands. Student turns the water to the preferred temperature and wets their hands. Student applies the soap to their hands and washes them with their hands pointed down. Student scrubs for 40–60 seconds and includes palm, between fingers, fingernails, and dorsum of hands. Student rinses hands with hands pointed down. Student dries their hands with a paper towel, uses a paper towel to turn off the water, and then disposes of the paper towel in the trash.	☐	☐	☐
	6	The student places the patient in the correct position for support, comfort, and access to body area necessary for data collection/intervention.	☐	☐	☐
Skill Performance	7	The student correctly performs **Sit to Stand Transfer**:			
		Student cues patient to scoot to the edge of the chair/bed and instructs them to position their feet so they are underneath patient (flat on the floor).	☐	☐	☐
		Student instructs patient to lean forward (nose over toes) and push from the chair/bed with one or both extremities, guarding and assisting as needed.	☐	☐	☐
	8	The student correctly performs **Stand to Sit Transfer**:			
		Student instructs patient to back up to the chair/bed until they feel the seat on the back of their legs.	☐	☐	☐
		Student instructs patient to reach back with one or both hands while leaning forward to slowly lower the buttocks toward the surface, guarding and assisting as needed. Student cues patient to lower to the surface slowly and controlled.	☐	☐	☐

⚐ = Critical Safety Element/Professionalism. If a student is unable to complete a flagged step without cueing, they will need to return at another time to redo the check-off. All other steps can be cued.

	9	The student correctly performs **Stand Pivot Transfer**:			
		Student positions the wheelchair so that it is parallel or at a 45-degree angle to the transfer surface. Transfers toward patient's stronger side.	☐	☐	☐
		Student locks the wheelchair brakes and removes the leg rests.	☐	☐	☐
		Student applies a gait belt to patient.	☐	☐	☐
		Student cues patient to scoot to the edge of the chair/bed and instructs them to position their feet so they are underneath patient (flat on the floor). Student assists as necessary.	☐	☐	☐
		Student instructs patient to lean forward (nose over toes) and push from the chair/bed with one or both extremities, guarding and assisting as needed.	☐	☐	☐
	⚐	Once patient is standing, student allows patient to gain their balance before instructing them to move their feet. **Do not allow patient to reach around your neck for support. If they are unsteady, cue them to reach for your forearms for support.**	☐	☐	☐
		Student instructs patient to back up to the chair/bed until they feel the seat on the back of their legs.	☐	☐	☐
		Student instructs patient to reach back with one or both hands while leaning forward to slowly lower the buttocks toward the surface, guarding and assisting as needed. Student cues patient to lower to the surface slowly and controlled.	☐	☐	☐
		Once patient is seated, student ensures they are safe before walking away.	☐	☐	☐
	10	The student correctly performs **Squat Pivot Transfer**:			
		Student positions the wheelchair so it is parallel or at a 45-degree angle to the transfer surface. Transfers toward patient's stronger side.	☐	☐	☐
		Student locks the wheelchair brakes and removes the leg rests.	☐	☐	☐
		Student applies a gait belt to patient.	☐	☐	☐
		Standing in front of patient, student cues patient to scoot to the edge of the chair/bed and instructs them to position their feet so they are underneath patient (flat on the floor). Student assists as necessary.	☐	☐	☐
		Student then assists patient with standing, but patient maintains a squat/bent knee position.	☐	☐	☐
		Patient pivots and sits on the other surface. Student assists as necessary.	☐	☐	☐
		Once patient is seated, student ensures they are safe before walking away.	☐	☐	☐

⚐ = Critical Safety Element/Professionalism. If a student is unable to complete a flagged step without cueing, they will need to return at another time to redo the check-off. All other steps can be cued.

	11	The student correctly performs **Slide Board Transfer**:			
		Student positions the wheelchair so it is parallel and as close as possible to the transfer surface. Transfers toward patient's stronger side.	☐	☐	☐
		Student locks the wheelchair brakes and removes the leg rests.	☐	☐	☐
		Student applies a gait belt to patient.	☐	☐	☐
		Student cues patient to lean away from the transfer side and slide the board under the buttocks so it is secure and will not move during the transfer. The other end of the board should be on the transfer surface. Student assists as necessary.	☐	☐	☐
		Student cues patient to lean forward and use both upper extremities to lift and move the buttocks across the board. Reminds patient not to wrap their fingers under the board or they will be pinched. Student assists as necessary.	☐	☐	☐
		Student guards and assist patient as needed until patient is completely on the new surface.	☐	☐	☐
		Student asks patient to lean away from the board so it can be removed from under the buttocks. Once patient is seated, student ensures they are safe before walking away.	☐	☐	☐
Post-Skill	12	The student washes their hands post–skill performance:			
		Student removes all jewelry from their wrists and hands. Student turns the water to the preferred temperature and wets their hands. Student applies the soap to their hands and washes them with their hands pointed down. Student scrubs for 40–60 seconds and includes palm, between fingers, fingernails, and dorsum of hands. Student rinses hands with hands pointed down. Student dries their hands with a paper towel, uses a paper towel to turn off the water, and then disposes of the paper towel in the trash.	☐	☐	☐
	13	The student verbalizes that they will document their session in the note.	☐	☐	☐
Other	14 ⚑	The student has optimal body mechanics during performance of the skill.	☐	☐	☐
	15 ⚑	The student uses appropriate therapeutic touch.	☐	☐	☐
	16	The student is able to complete the check-off in the time allotted.	☐	☐	☐
Communication	17	The student uses language the patient can understand.	☐	☐	☐
	18	The student listens actively to the patient during the session.	☐	☐	☐
	19	The student ensures the patient understands instructions by having the patient teach back or demonstrate.	☐	☐	☐
	20 ⚑	The student demonstrates confidence and provides the patient with clear instruction and cueing.	☐	☐	☐

Peer Name (Printed)		Peer Signature		Date of Peer Review	
Instructor Name (Printed and Signature)	By signing this skills checklist, I am declaring this student competent in the skill described above.			Date of Instructor Review	
NOTES					

⚑ = Critical Safety Element/Professionalism. If a student is unable to complete a flagged step without cueing, they will need to return at another time to redo the check-off. All other steps can be cued.

Student Name: _____

Skill		Functional Training: Handling Techniques			
Source		Lazaro RT, Umphred DA. *Umphred's Neurorehabilitation for the Physical Therapist Assistant.* 3rd ed. SLACK Incorporated; 2021.	**Check When Completed**		
			Self	Peer	Instructor
Student Introduction and Consent	1 ⚑	The student introduces themself to the patient. Must include that they are a **student** PTA and list the school's name.	☐	☐	☐
	2 ⚑	The student verifies the patient's identity. Must use at least 2 patient identifiers (name, date of birth).	☐	☐	☐
	3 ⚑	The student gains consent: • Speaks with the patient about their status (acquires relevant information) • Educates the patient on intended data collection/intervention and goals for the session • Gains permission to perform said data collection/intervention	☐	☐	☐
Student, Patient, and Supply Preparation	4 ⚑	The student gathers supplies and prepares treatment area (cleans equipment, checks for safety hazards, ensures all equipment is functional and appropriate).	☐	☐	☐
	5	The student washes their hands:			
		Student removes all jewelry from their wrists and hands. Student turns the water to the preferred temperature and wets their hands. Student applies the soap to their hands and washes them with their hands pointed down. Student scrubs for 40–60 seconds and includes palm, between fingers, fingernails, and dorsum of hands. Student rinses hands with hands pointed down. Student dries their hands with a paper towel, uses a paper towel to turn off the water, and then disposes of the paper towel in the trash.	☐	☐	☐
	6	The student places the patient in the correct position for support, comfort, and access to body area necessary for data collection/intervention.	☐	☐	☐
Skill Performance	7	The student correctly guides the patient during **Rolling From Supine to Sidelying** using proper handling:			
		To roll right, student will use the left leg/foot as the point of contact. Student initially handles the leg into flexion, slight abduction, and external rotation.	☐	☐	☐
		Student then controls the pelvis at the hip, using the entire leg while moving the leg toward the desired side. Patient's trunk follows through a body-on-head or body-on-body righting reaction.	☐	☐	☐
	8	The student correctly guides the patient during **Sidelying to Sitting** using proper handling:			
		While patient is in sidelying, student applies pressure to patient's topside anterior iliac crest in a downward and posterior direction to guide the topside hip into sitting.	☐	☐	☐
		Student assists the patient's upper body and head to vertical as needed by supporting patient from the back, under the bottom side arm and head.	☐	☐	☐
	9	The student correctly guides the patient during **Sitting** using proper handling:			
		Once patient is in sitting, student can support them from behind while sitting on an exercise ball (or sitting in half-kneel position). In this position, student can assist patient in various weight-shifting and reaching activities.	☐	☐	☐

⚑ = Critical Safety Element/Professionalism. If a student is unable to complete a flagged step without cueing, they will need to return at another time to redo the check-off. All other steps can be cued.

	10	The student correctly guides the patient during **Sit to Stand** using proper handling:			
		Student places seated patient facing a high/low mat.	☐	☐	☐
		Student brings patient forward in the chair and places their upper extremities over a medium-sized ball that is placed on the mat.	☐	☐	☐
		Student brings patient forward over the ball as the ball rolls onto the mat to bring their center of gravity over their feet.	☐	☐	☐
		Student then uses the high/low mat control device to raise the mat. The mat will bring patient to standing.	☐	☐	☐
		Student then stands behind patient to provide support while practicing weight-shifting activities.	☐	☐	☐
Post-Skill	11	The student washes their hands post–skill performance:			
		Student removes all jewelry from their wrists and hands. Student turns the water to the preferred temperature and wets their hands. Student applies the soap to their hands and washes them with their hands pointed down. Student scrubs for 40–60 seconds and includes palm, between fingers, fingernails, and dorsum of hands. Student rinses hands with hands pointed down. Student dries their hands with a paper towel, uses a paper towel to turn off the water, and then disposes of the paper towel in the trash.	☐	☐	☐
	12	The student verbalizes that they will document their session in the note.	☐	☐	☐
Other	13 ⚑	The student has optimal body mechanics during performance of the skill.	☐	☐	☐
	14 ⚑	The student uses appropriate therapeutic touch.	☐	☐	☐
	15	The student is able to complete the check-off in the time allotted.	☐	☐	☐
Communication	16	The student uses language the patient can understand.	☐	☐	☐
	17	The student listens actively to the patient during the session.	☐	☐	☐
	18	The student ensures the patient understands instructions by having the patient teach back or demonstrate.	☐	☐	☐
	19 ⚑	The student demonstrates confidence and provides the patient with clear instruction and cueing.	☐	☐	☐

Peer Name (Printed)		Peer Signature		Date of Peer Review	
Instructor Name (Printed and Signature)	By signing this skills checklist, I am declaring this student competent in the skill described above.			Date of Instructor Review	
NOTES					

⚑ = Critical Safety Element/Professionalism. If a student is unable to complete a flagged step without cueing, they will need to return at another time to redo the check-off. All other steps can be cued.

Student Name: _____

Skill		Functional Training: Facilitation Techniques			
Source		Lazaro RT, Umphred DA. *Umphred's Neurorehabilitation for the Physical Therapist Assistant.* 3rd ed. SLACK Incorporated; 2021.	Check When Completed		
			Self	Peer	Instructor
Student Introduction and Consent	1 ⚐	The student introduces themself to the patient. Must include that they are a **student** PTA and list the school's name.	☐	☐	☐
	2 ⚐	The student verifies the patient's identity. Must use at least 2 patient identifiers (name, date of birth).	☐	☐	☐
	3 ⚐	The student gains consent: • Speaks with the patient about their status (acquires relevant information) • Educates the patient on intended data collection/intervention and goals for the session • Gains permission to perform said data collection/intervention	☐	☐	☐
Student, Patient, and Supply Preparation	4 ⚐	The student gathers supplies and prepares treatment area (cleans equipment, checks for safety hazards, ensures all equipment is functional and appropriate).	☐	☐	☐
	5	The student washes their hands:			
		Student removes all jewelry from their wrists and hands. Student turns the water to the preferred temperature and wets their hands. Student applies the soap to their hands and washes them with their hands pointed down. Student scrubs for 40–60 seconds and includes palm, between fingers, fingernails, and dorsum of hands. Student rinses hands with hands pointed down. Student dries their hands with a paper towel, uses a paper towel to turn off the water, and then disposes of the paper towel in the trash.	☐	☐	☐
	6	The student places the patient in the correct position for support, comfort, and access to body area necessary for data collection/intervention.	☐	☐	☐
Skill Performance	7	The student correctly performs **Rhythmic Initiation** on instructor-selected motion:			
		Student moves patient through the desired movement using passive range of motion.	☐	☐	☐
		Student moves patient through the desired movement using active assisted range of motion.	☐	☐	☐
		Student moves patient through the desired movement using active range of motion.	☐	☐	☐
		Student moves patient through the desired movement providing resistance through the range of motion.	☐	☐	☐
	8	The student correctly performs **Contract Relax/Hold Relax** on instructor-selected muscle group:			
		Contract relax: Patient contracts selected muscle group followed by a sustained passive stretch by student.	☐	☐	☐
		Hold relax: Student provides a passive stretch to the selected muscle group followed by an isometric contraction by patient.	☐	☐	☐
	9	The student correctly performs **Rhythmic Stabilization** on instructor-selected joint:			
		Patient holds a position while student applies manual resistance. No motion should occur from patient.	☐	☐	☐
		Patient resists student's movements. Student holds this resistance and then switches to the alternate pattern, again with patient holding.	☐	☐	☐
	10	The student correctly performs **Alternating Isometrics** on instructor-selected joint:			
		Patient holds position while student applies manual resistance to both sides of the joint. No motion should occur from patient.	☐	☐	☐
		Patient resists student's movements. Student holds this resistance and then switches to the alternate pattern, again with patient holding.	☐	☐	☐

⚐ = Critical Safety Element/Professionalism. If a student is unable to complete a flagged step without cueing, they will need to return at another time to redo the check-off. All other steps can be cued.

	11	The student washes their hands post–skill performance:			
Post-Skill		Student removes all jewelry from their wrists and hands. Student turns the water to the preferred temperature and wets their hands. Student applies the soap to their hands and washes them with their hands pointed down. Student scrubs for 40–60 seconds and includes palm, between fingers, fingernails, and dorsum of hands. Student rinses hands with hands pointed down. Student dries their hands with a paper towel, uses a paper towel to turn off the water, and then disposes of the paper towel in the trash.	☐	☐	☐
	12	The student verbalizes that they will document their session in the note.	☐	☐	☐
Other	13 ⚑	The student has optimal body mechanics during performance of the skill.	☐	☐	☐
	14 ⚑	The student uses appropriate therapeutic touch.	☐	☐	☐
	15	The student is able to complete the check-off in the time allotted.	☐	☐	☐
Communication	16	The student uses language the patient can understand.	☐	☐	☐
	17	The student listens actively to the patient during the session.	☐	☐	☐
	18	The student ensures the patient understands instructions by having the patient teach back or demonstrate.	☐	☐	☐
	19 ⚑	The student demonstrates confidence and provides the patient with clear instruction and cueing.	☐	☐	☐

Peer Name (Printed)		Peer Signature		Date of Peer Review	
Instructor Name (Printed and Signature)	By signing this skills checklist, I am declaring this student competent in the skill described above.			Date of Instructor Review	
NOTES					

⚑ = Critical Safety Element/Professionalism. If a student is unable to complete a flagged step without cueing, they will need to return at another time to redo the check-off. All other steps can be cued.

Student Name: _____

Skill		Functional Training: Gait Patterns			
Source		Memolo J. *Procedures and Patient Care for the Physical Therapist Assistant.* SLACK Incorporated; 2019.	**Check When Completed**		
			Self	Peer	Instructor
Student Introduction and Consent	1 ⚑	The student introduces themself to the patient. Must include that they are a **student** PTA and list the school's name.	☐	☐	☐
	2 ⚑	The student verifies the patient's identity. Must use at least 2 patient identifiers (name, date of birth).	☐	☐	☐
	3 ⚑	The student gains consent: • Speaks with the patient about their status (acquires relevant information) • Educates the patient on intended data collection/intervention and goals for the session • Gains permission to perform said data collection/intervention	☐	☐	☐
Student, Patient, and Supply Preparation	4 ⚑	The student gathers supplies and prepares treatment area (cleans equipment, checks for safety hazards, ensures all equipment is functional and appropriate).	☐	☐	☐
	5	The student washes their hands:			
		Student removes all jewelry from their wrists and hands. Student turns the water to the preferred temperature and wets their hands. Student applies the soap to their hands and washes them with their hands pointed down. Student scrubs for 40–60 seconds and includes palm, between fingers, fingernails, and dorsum of hands. Student rinses hands with hands pointed down. Student dries their hands with a paper towel, uses a paper towel to turn off the water, and then disposes of the paper towel in the trash.	☐	☐	☐
	6	The student places the patient in the correct position for support, comfort, and access to body area necessary for data collection/intervention.	☐	☐	☐
	7	The student applies gait belt safely and securely to the patient.	☐	☐	☐
Skill Performance	8	The student correctly **Confirms the Fit of the Assistive Device**:			
		Walkers: Student positions the walker so patient is standing inside. The handgrip should come to the greater trochanter or wrist crease. When patient grasps the handgrips, elbow flexion should be 20–30 degrees.	☐	☐	☐
		Axillary crutches: Student positions the tips of the crutches 2 inches lateral and 4–6 inches anterior to patient's foot. The handgrip should come to the greater trochanter or wrist crease. When patient grasps the handgrips, the wrists should be straight and elbow flexion should be 20–30 degrees. There should be about 2 inches between the axilla and the top of the axillary rest (2–3 fingers).	☐	☐	☐
		Forearm crutches (Lofstrand crutches): Student positions the tips 2 inches lateral and 4–6 inches anterior to patient's foot. Patient's arms should be in the cuffs. When patient grasps the handgrips, elbow flexion should be 20–30 degrees. The cuff should be 1–1.5 inches below the olecranon process.	☐	☐	☐
		Canes: With patient in a standing or supine position, the handgrip should come to the greater trochanter or wrist crease. When patient grasps the handgrip, elbow flexion should be 0–30 degrees.	☐	☐	☐

⚑ = Critical Safety Element/Professionalism. If a student is unable to complete a flagged step without cueing, they will need to return at another time to redo the check-off. All other steps can be cued.

	9	The student correctly performs **3-Point Gait Pattern**:			
		Student describes which patients this gait pattern is best used for: *(Non–weight bearing, lower extremity amputation without prosthetic).*	☐	☐	☐
		Student describes which assistive device should be utilized: *(Axillary crutches, walker).*	☐	☐	☐
		Student instructs patient to advance the assistive device first, and then to step-to with the intact lower extremity.	☐	☐	☐
		Student guards and assists as necessary.	☐	☐	☐
	10	The student correctly performs **3-1 Gait Pattern and Modified 3-Point Gait Pattern**:			
		Student describes which patients this gait pattern is best used for: *(Partial weight bearing, touch down/toe touch weight bearing).*	☐	☐	☐
		Student describes which assistive device should be utilized: *(Axillary crutches, walker).*	☐	☐	☐
		Student instructs patient to advance the assistive device first.	☐	☐	☐
		Student instructs patient to advance the weight-bearing extremity and then quickly advance the intact lower extremity. (Alternatively, patient can advance the assistive device and the partial weight-bearing limb at the same time.)	☐	☐	☐
		Student guards and assists as necessary.	☐	☐	☐
	11	The student correctly performs **4-Point Gait Pattern**:			
		Student describes which patients this gait pattern is best used for: *(Weight bearing as tolerated to full weight bearing).*	☐	☐	☐
		Student describes which assistive device should be utilized: *(Axillary crutches, Lofstrand crutches).*	☐	☐	☐
		Student instructs patient to advance one assistive device and then advance the opposite lower extremity, not simultaneously.	☐	☐	☐
		The pattern is repeated with the opposite device and limb.	☐	☐	☐
		Student guards and assists as necessary.	☐	☐	☐
	12	The student correctly performs **Modified 4-Point Gait Pattern**:			
		Student describes which patients this gait pattern is best used for: *(Weight bearing as tolerated to full weight bearing).*	☐	☐	☐
		Student describes which assistive device should be utilized: *(Cane, single crutch).*	☐	☐	☐
		Student instructs patient to use the device on the opposite side of the injury.	☐	☐	☐
		Student instructs patient to first advance the assistive device, then advance the affected lower extremity followed by the intact lower extremity.	☐	☐	☐
		Student guards and assists as necessary.	☐	☐	☐
	13	The student correctly performs **2-Point Gait Pattern**:			
		Student describes which patients this gait pattern is best used for: *(Weight bearing as tolerated to full weight bearing).*	☐	☐	☐
		Student describes which assistive device should be utilized: *(Axillary crutches, Lofstrand crutches, bilateral canes).*	☐	☐	☐
		Student instructs patient to first advance one assistive device and the opposite lower extremity simultaneously.	☐	☐	☐
		Student guards and assists as necessary.	☐	☐	☐

☐ = Critical Safety Element/Professionalism. If a student is unable to complete a flagged step without cueing, they will need to return at another time to redo the check-off. All other steps can be cued.

14	The student correctly performs **Modified 2-Point Gait Pattern**:			
	Student describes which patients this gait pattern is best used for: *(Weight bearing as tolerated to full weight bearing)*.	☐	☐	☐
	Student describes which assistive device should be utilized: *(Cane, single crutch, hemi-walker)*.	☐	☐	☐
	Student instructs patient to use the device on the opposite side of the injury.	☐	☐	☐
	Student instructs patient to simultaneously advance the assistive device and the affected limb, followed by the intact limb.	☐	☐	☐
	Student guards and assists as necessary.	☐	☐	☐
15	The student correctly **Negotiates a Curb With an Assistive Device**:			
	Ascending a curb with a walker: Student stands behind patient and instructs patient to step up close to the curb. Patient then lifts and places the walker on the higher surface. Student then instructs patient to step up with the stronger lower extremity followed by the weaker. Student guards and assists as necessary.	☐	☐	☐
	Descending a curb with a walker: Student stands in front of patient and instructs patient to step up close to the curb. Patient then lifts and places the walker on the lower surface. Student then instructs patient to step down with the weaker lower extremity followed by the stronger. Student guards and assists as necessary.	☐	☐	☐
	Ascending a curb with crutches and non–weight bearing status: Student stands behind patient and instructs patient to step up close to the curb. Patient then pushes on the crutches to lift up the intact leg, followed by bringing up the crutches. Student guards and assists as necessary.	☐	☐	☐
	Descending a curb with crutches and non–weight bearing status: Student stands in front of patient and instructs patient to step up close to the curb. Patient lowers the crutches first and then steps down with the intact leg. Student guards and assists as necessary.	☐	☐	☐
	Ascending a curb with crutches and partial weight bearing to full weight bearing status: Student stands behind patient and instructs them to step up close to the curb. Patient then pushes on the crutches to lift up the intact leg, followed by bringing up weaker leg and the crutches. Student guards and assists as necessary.	☐	☐	☐
	Descending a curb with crutches and partial weight bearing to full weight bearing status: Student stands in front of patient and instructs them to step up close to the curb. Patient lowers the crutches first and then steps down with the weaker leg followed by the stronger leg. Student guards and assists as necessary.	☐	☐	☐
	Ascending a curb with a cane: Student stands behind patient and instructs them to step up close to the curb. Patient advances the stronger leg first, followed by the cane, and then the weaker leg. Student guards and assists as necessary.	☐	☐	☐
	Descending a curb with a cane: Student stands in front of patient and instructs them to step up close to the curb. Patient lowers the weaker leg and the cane first, followed by the stronger leg. Student guards and assists as necessary.	☐	☐	☐

☐ = Critical Safety Element/Professionalism. If a student is unable to complete a flagged step without cueing, they will need to return at another time to redo the check-off. All other steps can be cued.

	16	The student correctly **Negotiates Stairs With an Assistive Device:**			
		Ascending stairs with a walker: Student stands behind patient and instructs them to step up close to the stairs. Patient then steps up with the intact lower extremity first. The affected limb will follow as patient also advances the walker. Student guards and assists as necessary.	☐	☐	☐
		Descending stairs with a walker: Student stands in front of patient and instructs them to step up close to the stairs. Patient then steps down with the affected limb while also lowering the walker to the next step, and then follows with the intact limb. Student guards and assists as necessary.	☐	☐	☐
		Ascending stairs with a cane: Student stands behind patient and instructs them to step up close to the stairs. Patient then steps up with the intact lower extremity first, followed by the cane, and then the affected lower extremity. Student guards and assists as necessary.	☐	☐	☐
		Descending stairs with a cane: Student stands in front of patient and instructs them to step up close to the stairs. Patient first advances the cane and then the affected lower extremity, followed by the unaffected lower extremity. Student guards and assists as necessary.	☐	☐	☐
		Ascending stairs with crutches and non–weight bearing status: Student stands behind patient and instructs them to step up close to the stairs. Patient then pushes on the crutches to lift the intact leg up. Patient lifts the crutches to the next step with the non–weight bearing leg flexed at the knee and behind so it will not catch on the step. Student guards and assists as necessary.	☐	☐	☐
		Descending stairs with crutches and non–weight bearing status: Student stands in front of patient and instructs them to step up close to the stairs. Patient descends by advancing the crutches down, followed by the unaffected lower extremity while keeping the affected lower extremity with the knee extended out in front to avoid catching on the step. Student guards and assists as necessary.	☐	☐	☐
		Ascending stairs with crutches and partial weight bearing to full weight bearing status: Student stands behind patient and instructs them to step up close to the stairs. Patient then pushes on the crutches to lift the intact leg up, followed by bringing up weaker leg and the crutches. Student guards and assists as necessary.	☐	☐	☐
		Descending a curb with crutches and partial weight bearing to full weight bearing status: Student stands in front of patient and instructs them to step up close to the stairs. Patient lowers the crutches first and then steps down with the weaker leg followed by the stronger leg. Student guards and assists as necessary.	☐	☐	☐
Post-Skill	17	The student washes their hands post–skill performance:			
		Student removes all jewelry from their wrists and hands. Student turns the water to the preferred temperature and wets their hands. Student applies the soap to their hands and washes them with their hands pointed down. Student scrubs for 40–60 seconds and includes palm, between fingers, fingernails, and dorsum of hands. Student rinses hands with hands pointed down. Student dries their hands with a paper towel, uses a paper towel to turn off the water, and then disposes of the paper towel in the trash.	☐	☐	☐
	18	The student verbalizes that they will document their session in the note.	☐	☐	☐
Other	19 ⚑	The student has optimal body mechanics during performance of the skill.	☐	☐	☐
	20 ⚑	The student uses appropriate therapeutic touch.	☐	☐	☐
	21	The student is able to complete the check-off in the time allotted.	☐	☐	☐

⚑ = Critical Safety Element/Professionalism. If a student is unable to complete a flagged step without cueing, they will need to return at another time to redo the check-off. All other steps can be cued.

Communication	22	The student uses language the patient can understand.	☐	☐	☐
	23	The student listens actively to the patient during the session.	☐	☐	☐
	24	The student ensures the patient understands instructions by having the patient teach back or demonstrate.	☐	☐	☐
	25 ⚑	The student demonstrates confidence and provides the patient with clear instruction and cueing.	☐	☐	☐

Peer Name (Printed)		**Peer Signature**		**Date of Peer Review**	
Instructor Name (Printed and Signature)	By signing this skills checklist, I am declaring this student competent in the skill described above.			**Date of Instructor Review**	
NOTES					

⚑ = Critical Safety Element/Professionalism. If a student is unable to complete a flagged step without cueing, they will need to return at another time to redo the check-off. All other steps can be cued.

Student Name: _____

Skill		Functional Training: Wheelchair Operation			
Source		Memolo J. *Procedures and Patient Care for the Physical Therapist Assistant.* SLACK Incorporated; 2019.	**Check When Completed**		
			Self	Peer	Instructor
Student Introduction and Consent	1 ⚑	The student introduces themself to the patient. Must include that they are a **student** PTA and list the school's name.	☐	☐	☐
	2 ⚑	The student verifies the patient's identity. Must use at least 2 patient identifiers (name, date of birth).	☐	☐	☐
	3 ⚑	The student gains consent: • Speaks with the patient about their status (acquires relevant information) • Educates the patient on intended data collection/intervention and goals for the session • Gains permission to perform said data collection/intervention	☐	☐	☐
Student, Patient, and Supply Preparation	4 ⚑	The student gathers supplies and prepares treatment area (cleans equipment, checks for safety hazards, ensures all equipment is functional and appropriate).	☐	☐	☐
	5	The student washes their hands:			
		Student removes all jewelry from their wrists and hands. Student turns the water to the preferred temperature and wets their hands. Student applies the soap to their hands and washes them with their hands pointed down. Student scrubs for 40–60 seconds and includes palm, between fingers, fingernails, and dorsum of hands. Student rinses hands with hands pointed down. Student dries their hands with a paper towel, uses a paper towel to turn off the water, and then disposes of the paper towel in the trash.	☐	☐	☐
	6	The student ensures that the wheelchair fits properly to the patient:			
		Seat height/leg length: Patient should be sitting with their feet on the footrests. Student should be able to place 2–3 fingers between patient's thigh and the seat. The bottom of the footrests should be 2 inches from the floor.	☐	☐	☐
		Seat depth: Patient should be seated back in the chair. Student should be able to place 2–3 fingers between the front edge of the seat and patient's popliteal folds.	☐	☐	☐
		Seat width: Student's hands should fit vertically between patient's hips and the chair's armrests.	☐	☐	☐
		Back height: Student should be able to fit 4 fingers (with hands held vertically) between the top of the back of the seat and the floor of patient's axilla.	☐	☐	☐
		Armrest height: Patient's shoulders should be level, the position of the trunk should be erect, and they should be able to rest their arms on the armrests with no change in posture.	☐	☐	☐

⚑ = Critical Safety Element/Professionalism. If a student is unable to complete a flagged step without cueing, they will need to return at another time to redo the check-off. All other steps can be cued.

Skill Performance	7	The student correctly teaches patient **Wheelchair Propulsion**:			
		To move forward: Student instructs patient to hold the drive wheels at the 12 o'clock position. Patient is to push forward with both arms at the same time with the same force.	☐	☐	☐
		To move backward: Student instructs patient to hold the drive wheels at the 12 o'clock position. Patient is to push backward with both arms at the same time with the same force.	☐	☐	☐
		To turn: Student instructs patient to hold the drive wheels at the 12 o'clock position. Patient is to push forward on the opposite wheel of the direction they want to turn while simultaneously pulling back on the other wheel.	☐	☐	☐
		To ascend a curb forward: Student faces the wheelchair toward the curb and tips patient back onto the drive wheels using the tipping device. The caster wheels are placed up on the curb and student should lift the chair to put the drive wheels on the curb.	☐	☐	☐
		To ascend a curb backward: Student faces the wheelchair away from the curb and tips patient back onto the drive wheels using the tipping device. Student then carefully lifts the drive wheels onto the curb, pulls the chair back, and slowly lowers the chair until the caster wheels are placed up on the curb.	☐	☐	☐
		To descend a curb forward: Student faces the wheelchair toward the curb and tips patient back onto the drive wheels using the tipping device. Student then slowly lowers the wheelchair off the curb onto the lower surface and then carefully lowers caster wheels onto the surface.	☐	☐	☐
		To descend a curb backward: Student faces the wheelchair away from the curb. Student slowly lowers the drive wheels off the curb and then tips patient back onto the drive wheels using the tipping device. Student then backs up enough to allow the caster wheels to be lowered to the ground.	☐	☐	☐
		To ascend a ramp: Student instructs patient to lean forward in the chair and push equally with both upper extremities.	☐	☐	☐
		To descend a ramp: Student instructs patient to lean back in the chair and use both upper extremities to provide friction on the drive wheels to slow the descent.	☐	☐	☐
Post-Skill	8	The student washes their hands post–skill performance:			
		Student removes all jewelry from their wrists and hands. Student turns the water to the preferred temperature and wets their hands. Student applies the soap to their hands and washes them with their hands pointed down. Student scrubs for 40–60 seconds and includes palm, between fingers, fingernails, and dorsum of hands. Student rinses hands with hands pointed down. Student dries their hands with a paper towel, uses a paper towel to turn off the water, and then disposes of the paper towel in the trash.	☐	☐	☐
	9	The student verbalizes that they will document their session in the note.	☐	☐	☐

☐ = Critical Safety Element/Professionalism. If a student is unable to complete a flagged step without cueing, they will need to return at another time to redo the check-off. All other steps can be cued.

Other	10 ⚑	The student has optimal body mechanics during performance of the skill.	☐	☐	☐
	11 ⚑	The student uses appropriate therapeutic touch.	☐	☐	☐
	12	The student is able to complete the check-off in the time allotted.	☐	☐	☐
Communication	13	The student uses language the patient can understand.	☐	☐	☐
	14	The student listens actively to the patient during the session.	☐	☐	☐
	15	The student ensures the patient understands instructions by having the patient teach back or demonstrate.	☐	☐	☐
	16 ⚑	The student demonstrates confidence and provides the patient with clear instruction and cueing.	☐	☐	☐

Peer Name (Printed)		Peer Signature		Date of Peer Review	
Instructor Name (Printed and Signature)	By signing this skills checklist, I am declaring this student competent in the skill described above.			Date of Instructor Review	
NOTES					

⚑ = Critical Safety Element/Professionalism. If a student is unable to complete a flagged step without cueing, they will need to return at another time to redo the check-off. All other steps can be cued.

Student Name: _____

Skill		Functional Training: Lifting Techniques			
Source		Memolo J. *Procedures and Patient Care for the Physical Therapist Assistant.* SLACK Incorporated; 2019.	Check When Completed		
			Self	Peer	Instructor
Student Introduction and Consent	1 ⚑	The student introduces themself to the patient. Must include that they are a **student** PTA and list the school's name.	☐	☐	☐
	2 ⚑	The student verifies the patient's identity. Must use at least 2 patient identifiers (name, date of birth).	☐	☐	☐
	3 ⚑	The student gains consent: • Speaks with the patient about their status (acquires relevant information) • Educates the patient on intended data collection/intervention and goals for the session • Gains permission to perform said data collection/intervention	☐	☐	☐
Student, Patient, and Supply Preparation	4 ⚑	The student gathers supplies and prepares treatment area (cleans equipment, checks for safety hazards, ensures all equipment is functional and appropriate).	☐	☐	☐
	5	The student washes their hands:			
		Student removes all jewelry from their wrists and hands. Student turns the water to the preferred temperature and wets their hands. Student applies the soap to their hands and washes them with their hands pointed down. Student scrubs for 40–60 seconds and includes palm, between fingers, fingernails, and dorsum of hands. Student rinses hands with hands pointed down. Student dries their hands with a paper towel, uses a paper towel to turn off the water, and then disposes of the paper towel in the trash.	☐	☐	☐
	6	The student places the patient in the correct position for support, comfort, and access to body area necessary for data collection/intervention.	☐	☐	☐
	7	The student educates the patient on basic lifting principles: *(Get close to the item to be lifted Lower your center of gravity Widen your base of support Maintain lumbar lordosis Avoid twisting and flexing the spine Bend at the hips, not the waist).*	☐	☐	☐
Skill Performance	8	The student correctly teaches the patient to perform a **Deep Squat Lift**:			
		Student instructs patient to place their feet in a parallel position straddling the object to be lifted.	☐	☐	☐
		Student instructs patient to lower their hips below the level of their knees.	☐	☐	☐
		Student instructs patient to grasp the object with both hands, pull it close to their body, and then stand. Reminds patient to maintain lumbar lordosis.	☐	☐	☐
		Student observes patient performing the deep squat lift and corrects any errors.	☐	☐	☐
	9	The student correctly teaches the patient to perform a **Power Lift**:			
		Student instructs patient to place their feet in a parallel position behind the object to be lifted.	☐	☐	☐
		Student instructs patient to lower their hips but not past the level of their knees.	☐	☐	☐
		Student instructs patient to grasp the object with both hands, pull it close to their body, and then stand. Reminds patient to maintain lumbar lordosis.	☐	☐	☐
		Student observes patient performing the power lift and corrects any errors.	☐	☐	☐

⚑ = Critical Safety Element/Professionalism. If a student is unable to complete a flagged step without cueing, they will need to return at another time to redo the check-off. All other steps can be cued.

	10	The student correctly teaches the patient to perform a **Straight Leg Lift**:			
		Student informs patient that this lift is ideal for getting items near waist level.	☐	☐	☐
		Student instructs patient to place their feet in a parallel position near the object to be lifted.	☐	☐	☐
		Student instructs patient to flex their knees and bend at the hips slightly.	☐	☐	☐
		Student instructs patient to grasp the object with both hands, pull it close to their body, and then stand. Student reminds patient to maintain lumbar lordosis.	☐	☐	☐
		Student observes patient performing the straight leg lift and corrects any errors.	☐	☐	☐
	11	The student correctly teaches the patient to perform a **Straight Leg Stance Lift**:			
		Student informs patient that this lift is only used with lightweight items.	☐	☐	☐
		Student instructs patient to place their feet in a parallel position near the object to be lifted.	☐	☐	☐
		Student instructs patient to shift their weight to one leg with their knee and hip slightly flexed, while the other leg is kicked behind them, keeping that knee straight.	☐	☐	☐
		Student instructs patient to flex at the hips while using one extremity to reach for and retrieve the item before returning to vertical.	☐	☐	☐
		Student observes patient performing the straight leg stance lift and corrects any errors.	☐	☐	☐
	12	The student correctly teaches the patient to perform a **Half-Kneeling Lift**:			
		Student instructs patient to stand near the item to be lifted and lower down to one knee with the other knee and hip flexed at 90 degrees.	☐	☐	☐
		Student instructs patient to grasp the item and pull it close to their body (propping it on the 90–90 knee).	☐	☐	☐
		Student instructs patient to return to standing while still holding the item close to the body. Student reminds patient to maintain lumbar lordosis.	☐	☐	☐
		Student observes patient performing the half-kneeling lift and corrects any errors.	☐	☐	☐
		Student explains that this lift is beneficial for patients with poor upper extremity strength, but it would be difficult for someone with poor balance or painful knees.	☐	☐	☐
	13	The student correctly teaches the patient to perform a **Traditional Lift**:			
		Student instructs patient to place their feet in an anterior-posterior position on either side of the object to be lifted.	☐	☐	☐
		Student instructs patient to lower their hips below the level of their knees.	☐	☐	☐
		Student instructs patient to grasp the object with both hands, pull it close to their body, and then stand. Student reminds patient to maintain lumbar lordosis.	☐	☐	☐
		Student observes patient performing the traditional lift and corrects any errors.	☐	☐	☐
	14	The student correctly teaches the patient to perform a **Stoop Lift**:			
		Student informs patient that this lift is good for items below the waist that can be lifted without squatting (briefcase, backpack, purse, etc).	☐	☐	☐
		Student instructs patient to place their feet in a parallel position next to the object to be lifted.	☐	☐	☐
		Student instructs patient to flex at the hips and knees while reaching for the item with one upper extremity. Patient grasps the object and returns to standing, avoiding lateral bending or twisting of the trunk. Student reminds patient to maintain lumbar lordosis.	☐	☐	☐
		Student observes patient performing the stoop lift and corrects any errors.	☐	☐	☐

⌐☐ = Critical Safety Element/Professionalism. If a student is unable to complete a flagged step without cueing, they will need to return at another time to redo the check-off. All other steps can be cued.

Post-Skill	15	The student washes their hands post–skill performance:			
		Student removes all jewelry from their wrists and hands. Student turns the water to the preferred temperature and wets their hands. Student applies the soap to their hands and washes them with their hands pointed down. Student scrubs for 40–60 seconds and includes palm, between fingers, fingernails, and dorsum of hands. Student rinses hands with hands pointed down. Student dries their hands with a paper towel, uses a paper towel to turn off the water, and then disposes of the paper towel in the trash.	☐	☐	☐
	16	The student verbalizes that they will document their session in the note.	☐	☐	☐
Other	17 ⚑	The student has optimal body mechanics during performance of the skill.	☐	☐	☐
	18 ⚑	The student uses appropriate therapeutic touch.	☐	☐	☐
	19	The student is able to complete the check-off in the time allotted.	☐	☐	☐
Communication	20	The student uses language the patient can understand.	☐	☐	☐
	21	The student listens actively to the patient during the session.	☐	☐	☐
	22	The student ensures the patient understands instructions by having the patient teach back or demonstrate.	☐	☐	☐
	23 ⚑	The student demonstrates confidence and provides the patient with clear instruction and cueing.	☐	☐	☐

Peer Name (Printed)		Peer Signature		Date of Peer Review	
Instructor Name (Printed and Signature)	By signing this skills checklist, I am declaring this student competent in the skill described above.			Date of Instructor Review	
NOTES					

⚑ = Critical Safety Element/Professionalism. If a student is unable to complete a flagged step without cueing, they will need to return at another time to redo the check-off. All other steps can be cued.

Chapter 14

Manual Therapy

Larson T. *Entry-Level Skill Checklists for
Physical Therapist Assistant Students* (pp 161-168).
© 2023 Taylor & Francis Group.

Student Name: _____

Skill		Manual Therapy: Soft Tissue Mobilization			
Source		Memolo J. *Therapeutic Agents for the Physical Therapist Assistant.* SLACK Incorporated; 2022.	Check When Completed		
			Self	Peer	Instructor
Student Introduction and Consent	1 ⚑	The student introduces themself to the patient. Must include that they are a **student** PTA and list the school's name.	☐	☐	☐
	2 ⚑	The student verifies the patient's identity. Must use at least 2 patient identifiers (name, date of birth).	☐	☐	☐
	3 ⚑	The student gains consent: • Speaks with the patient about their status (acquires relevant information) • Educates the patient on intended data collection/intervention and goals for the session • Gains permission to perform said data collection/intervention	☐	☐	☐
Student, Patient, and Supply Preparation	4 ⚑	The student gathers supplies and prepares treatment area (cleans equipment, checks for safety hazards, ensures all equipment is functional and appropriate).	☐	☐	☐
	5	The student washes their hands:			
		Student removes all jewelry from their wrists and hands. Student turns the water to the preferred temperature and wets their hands. Student applies the soap to their hands and washes them with their hands pointed down. Student scrubs for 40–60 seconds and includes palm, between fingers, fingernails, and dorsum of hands. Student rinses hands with hands pointed down. Student dries their hands with a paper towel, uses a paper towel to turn off the water, and then disposes of the paper towel in the trash.	☐	☐	☐
	6	The student places the patient in the correct position for support, comfort, and access to body area necessary for data collection/intervention.	☐	☐	☐
Skill Performance	7	The student correctly applies **Effleurage**:			
		Student determines that patient does not have any contraindications.	☐	☐	☐
		Patient is positioned and draped to provide warmth, protect patient's clothes, prevent pressure build-up, and access the body part(s) required.	☐	☐	☐
		Student uses the appropriate type and amount of lubricant.	☐	☐	☐
		Student performs light, gliding strokes using their full hand and follows the muscle fibers moving toward the heart.	☐	☐	☐
	8	The student correctly applies **Petrissage**:			
		Student determines that patient does not have any contraindications.	☐	☐	☐
		Patient is positioned and draped to provide warmth, protect patient's clothes, prevent pressure build-up, and access the body part(s) required.	☐	☐	☐
		Student uses the appropriate type and amount of lubricant.	☐	☐	☐
		Student performs light, kneading strokes using their full hand and follows the muscle fibers moving toward the heart.	☐	☐	☐

⚑ = Critical Safety Element/Professionalism. If a student is unable to complete a flagged step without cueing, they will need to return at another time to redo the check-off. All other steps can be cued.

	9	The student correctly applies **Friction Massage**:			
		Student determines that patient does not have any contraindications.	☐	☐	☐
		Patient is positioned and draped to provide warmth, protect patient's clothes, prevent pressure build-up, and access the body part(s) required.	☐	☐	☐
		Student uses the appropriate type and amount of lubricant.	☐	☐	☐
		Student uses the fingertips, thumbs, or heel of the hand to supply sufficient pressure to the selected area.	☐	☐	☐
		Student applies deep pressure to the area and then makes small circular motions over the localized point. Student may also perform a transverse movement perpendicular to the tissue fibers.	☐	☐	☐
Post-Skill	10	The student washes their hands post–skill performance:			
		Student removes all jewelry from their wrists and hands. Student turns the water to the preferred temperature and wets their hands. Student applies the soap to their hands and washes them with their hands pointed down. Student scrubs for 40–60 seconds and includes palm, between fingers, fingernails, and dorsum of hands. Student rinses hands with hands pointed down. Student dries their hands with a paper towel, uses a paper towel to turn off the water, and then disposes of the paper towel in the trash.	☐	☐	☐
	11	The student verbalizes that they will document their session in the note.	☐	☐	☐
Other	12 ⚑	The student has optimal body mechanics during performance of the skill.	☐	☐	☐
	13 ⚑	The student uses appropriate therapeutic touch.	☐	☐	☐
	14	The student is able to complete the check-off in the time allotted.	☐	☐	☐
Communication	15	The student uses language the patient can understand.	☐	☐	☐
	16	The student listens actively to the patient during the session.	☐	☐	☐
	17	The student ensures the patient understands instructions by having the patient teach back or demonstrate.	☐	☐	☐
	18 ⚑	The student demonstrates confidence and provides the patient with clear instruction and cueing.	☐	☐	☐

Peer Name (Printed)		**Peer Signature**		**Date of Peer Review**	
Instructor Name (Printed and Signature)	By signing this skills checklist, I am declaring this student competent in the skill described above.			**Date of Instructor Review**	

NOTES	

⚑ = Critical Safety Element/Professionalism. If a student is unable to complete a flagged step without cueing, they will need to return at another time to redo the check-off. All other steps can be cued.

Student Name: _____

Skill		Manual Therapy: Joint Mobilization—Upper Quarter			
Source		Physical Therapy. Education. Redefined. PhysioU. Accessed September 14, 2022. https://www.physiou.health/	**Check When Completed**		
			Self	Peer	Instructor
Student Introduction and Consent	1 ⚑	The student introduces themself to the patient. Must include that they are a **student** PTA and list the school's name.	☐	☐	☐
	2 ⚑	The student verifies the patient's identity. Must use at least 2 patient identifiers (name, date of birth).	☐	☐	☐
	3 ⚑	The student gains consent: • Speaks with the patient about their status (acquires relevant information) • Educates the patient on intended data collection/intervention and goals for the session • Gains permission to perform said data collection/intervention	☐	☐	☐
Student, Patient, and Supply Preparation	4 ⚑	The student gathers supplies and prepares treatment area (cleans equipment, checks for safety hazards, ensures all equipment is functional and appropriate).	☐	☐	☐
	5	The student washes their hands:			
		Student removes all jewelry from their wrists and hands. Student turns the water to the preferred temperature and wets their hands. Student applies the soap to their hands and washes them with their hands pointed down. Student scrubs for 40–60 seconds and includes palm, between fingers, fingernails, and dorsum of hands. Student rinses hands with hands pointed down. Student dries their hands with a paper towel, uses a paper towel to turn off the water, and then disposes of the paper towel in the trash.	☐	☐	☐
	6	The student places the patient in the correct position for support, comfort, and access to body area necessary for data collection/intervention.	☐	☐	☐
Skill Performance	7	The student correctly applies **Glenohumeral Joint Anterior Glide**:			
		Student determines that patient does not have any contraindications.	☐	☐	☐
		Patient is positioned in prone and draped to provide warmth and access the body part(s) required.	☐	☐	☐
		Student stabilizes the shoulder girdle with one hand and places their thenar eminence of mobilization hand on the posterior humeral head.	☐	☐	☐
		Student provides an anterior-directed force.	☐	☐	☐
	8	The student correctly applies **Glenohumeral Joint Posterior Glide**:			
		Student determines that patient does not have any contraindications.	☐	☐	☐
		Patient is positioned in prone with the arm in the open pack position, draped to provide warmth and access the body part(s) required.	☐	☐	☐
		Student stabilizes patient's hand in student's axillary region.	☐	☐	☐
		Student grasps patient's distal humerus with the nonmobilization hand and places the thenar eminence of the mobilization hand over the anterior head of the humerus.	☐	☐	☐
		Student provides a posterior-directed force.	☐	☐	☐
	9	The student correctly applies **Radiocarpal Dorsal Glide**:			
		Student determines that patient does not have any contraindications.	☐	☐	☐
		Patient is positioned in supine or seated with forearm supported on the table with wrist in supination.	☐	☐	☐
		Student stabilizes patient's distal radius and ulnar with one hand and stabilizes the proximal carpal row with the other.	☐	☐	☐
		Student provides a downward force to the first carpal row with a grade 1 traction.	☐	☐	☐

⚑ = Critical Safety Element/Professionalism. If a student is unable to complete a flagged step without cueing, they will need to return at another time to redo the check-off. All other steps can be cued.

	10	The student correctly applies **Radiocarpal Volar Glide**:			
		Student determines that patient does not have any contraindications.	☐	☐	☐
		Patient is positioned in supine or seated with forearm supported on the table with wrist in pronation.	☐	☐	☐
		Student stabilizes patient's distal radius and ulnar with one hand and stabilizes the proximal carpal row with the other.	☐	☐	☐
		Student provides a downward force to the first carpal row with a grade 1 traction.	☐	☐	☐
Post-Skill	11	The student washes their hands post–skill performance:			
		Student removes all jewelry from their wrists and hands. Student turns the water to the preferred temperature and wets their hands. Student applies the soap to their hands and washes them with their hands pointed down. Student scrubs for 40–60 seconds and includes palm, between fingers, fingernails, and dorsum of hands. Student rinses hands with hands pointed down. Student dries their hands with a paper towel, uses a paper towel to turn off the water, and then disposes of the paper towel in the trash.	☐	☐	☐
	12	The student verbalizes that they will document their session in the note.	☐	☐	☐
Other	13 ⚑	The student has optimal body mechanics during performance of the skill.	☐	☐	☐
	14 ⚑	The student uses appropriate therapeutic touch.	☐	☐	☐
	15	The student is able to complete the check-off in the time allotted.	☐	☐	☐
Communication	16	The student uses language the patient can understand.	☐	☐	☐
	17	The student listens actively to the patient during the session.	☐	☐	☐
	18	The student ensures the patient understands instructions by having the patient teach back or demonstrate.	☐	☐	☐
	19 ⚑	The student demonstrates confidence and provides the patient with clear instruction and cueing.	☐	☐	☐

Peer Name (Printed)		**Peer Signature**		**Date of Peer Review**	
Instructor Name (Printed and Signature)	By signing this skills checklist, I am declaring this student competent in the skill described above.			**Date of Instructor Review**	
NOTES					

⚑ = Critical Safety Element/Professionalism. If a student is unable to complete a flagged step without cueing, they will need to return at another time to redo the check-off. All other steps can be cued.

Student Name: _____

Skill		Manual Therapy: Joint Mobilization—Lower Quarter			
Source		Physical Therapy. Education. Redefined. PhysioU. Accessed September 14, 2022. https://www.physiou.health/	**Check When Completed**		
			Self	Peer	Instructor
Student Introduction and Consent	1 ⚑	The student introduces themself to the patient. Must include that they are a **student** PTA and list the school's name.	☐	☐	☐
	2 ⚑	The student verifies the patient's identity. Must use at least 2 patient identifiers (name, date of birth).	☐	☐	☐
	3 ⚑	The student gains consent: • Speaks with the patient about their status (acquires relevant information) • Educates the patient on intended data collection/intervention and goals for the session • Gains permission to perform said data collection/intervention	☐	☐	☐
Student, Patient, and Supply Preparation	4 ⚑	The student gathers supplies and prepares treatment area (cleans equipment, checks for safety hazards, ensures all equipment is functional and appropriate).	☐	☐	☐
	5	The student washes their hands:			
		Student removes all jewelry from their wrists and hands. Student turns the water to the preferred temperature and wets their hands. Student applies the soap to their hands and washes them with their hands pointed down. Student scrubs for 40–60 seconds and includes palm, between fingers, fingernails, and dorsum of hands. Student rinses hands with hands pointed down. Student dries their hands with a paper towel, uses a paper towel to turn off the water, and then disposes of the paper towel in the trash.	☐	☐	☐
	6	The student places the patient in the correct position for support, comfort, and access to body area necessary for data collection/intervention.	☐	☐	☐
Skill Performance	7	The student correctly applies **Hip Longitudinal Distraction**:			
		Student determines that patient does not have any contraindications.	☐	☐	☐
		Patient is positioned in supine and draped to provide warmth and access the body part(s) required.	☐	☐	☐
		Student grasps patient's ankle and gently brings patient's hip into the open packed position (30 degrees flexion, 30 degrees abduction, and slight external rotation).	☐	☐	☐
		With hands grasped around patient's ankle, student gently leans back, keeping elbows straight, and provides a gentle distraction or a grade 1 or grade 2 oscillation.	☐	☐	☐
	8	The student correctly applies **Hip Posterior Glide**:			
		Student determines that patient does not have any contraindications.	☐	☐	☐
		Patient is positioned in supine with involved leg crossed over uninvolved leg with foot flat on table.	☐	☐	☐
		Student interlocks fingers and places their hands over patient's anterior knee and braces patient's knee against their sternum.	☐	☐	☐
		Student applies an axial anterior to posterior force through the femur, toward the hip joint.	☐	☐	☐

⚑ = Critical Safety Element/Professionalism. If a student is unable to complete a flagged step without cueing, they will need to return at another time to redo the check-off. All other steps can be cued.

	9	The student correctly applies **Tibiofemoral Anterior Glide**:			
		Student determines that patient does not have any contraindications.	☐	☐	☐
		Patient is positioned in prone with knees off end of table with a small towel roll under the distal femur of the involved leg.	☐	☐	☐
		Student extends the involved knee to its available range and stabilizes the involved ankle with the caudal hand.	☐	☐	☐
		Student places the cephalad hand on the posterior surface of the proximal tibia.	☐	☐	☐
		Student provides an anterior force through cephalad hand by shifting body weight through a fully extended elbow.	☐	☐	☐
	10	The student correctly applies **Tibiofemoral Traction Mobilization**:			
		Student determines that patient does not have any contraindications.	☐	☐	☐
		Patient is positioned in a seated position at the edge of the table.	☐	☐	☐
		Student stabilizes patient's distal tibia between the therapist's knees and raises the plinth to provide an inferior tibiofemoral traction force.	☐	☐	☐
		Student grasps the superior aspect of the tibia with both hands and provides a posterior or anterior tibiofemoral glide.	☐	☐	☐
	11	The student correctly applies **Talocrural Posterior Glide**:			
		Student determines that patient does not have any contraindications.	☐	☐	☐
		Patient is positioned in a supine position with heel off edge of the table.	☐	☐	☐
		Student places their thumbs or 2nd metacarpal head on the dorsal surface of the talus.	☐	☐	☐
		Student takes up tissue slack and applies a posterior-directed force at the talus.	☐	☐	☐
	12	The student correctly applies **Talocrural Anterior Glide**:			
		Student determines that patient does not have any contraindications.	☐	☐	☐
		Patient is positioned in a prone position with heel off edge of the table.	☐	☐	☐
		Student places a towel underneath the anterior part of the distal tibia to cushion the leg against the table.	☐	☐	☐
		With one hand, student grasps the anterior portion of the talus and applies an anterior glide pulling force. With the other hand, student provides an anterior-directed mobilization through the calcaneus.	☐	☐	☐
Post-Skill	13	The student washes their hands post–skill performance:			
		Student removes all jewelry from their wrists and hands. Student turns the water to the preferred temperature and wets their hands. Student applies the soap to their hands and washes them with their hands pointed down. Student scrubs for 40–60 seconds and includes palm, between fingers, fingernails, and dorsum of hands. Student rinses hands with hands pointed down. Student dries their hands with a paper towel, uses a paper towel to turn off the water, and then disposes of the paper towel in the trash.	☐	☐	☐
	14	The student verbalizes that they will document their session in the note.	☐	☐	☐

☐ = Critical Safety Element/Professionalism. If a student is unable to complete a flagged step without cueing, they will need to return at another time to redo the check-off. All other steps can be cued.

Other	15 ⚑	The student has optimal body mechanics during performance of the skill.		☐	☐	☐
	16 ⚑	The student uses appropriate therapeutic touch.		☐	☐	☐
	17	The student is able to complete the check-off in the time allotted.		☐	☐	☐
Communication	18	The student uses language the patient can understand.		☐	☐	☐
	19	The student listens actively to the patient during the session.		☐	☐	☐
	20	The student ensures the patient understands instructions by having the patient teach back or demonstrate.		☐	☐	☐
	21 ⚑	The student demonstrates confidence and provides the patient with clear instruction and cueing.		☐	☐	☐

Peer Name (Printed)		Peer Signature		Date of Peer Review	
Instructor Name (Printed and Signature)	By signing this skills checklist, I am declaring this student competent in the skill described above.			Date of Instructor Review	
NOTES					

⚑ = Critical Safety Element/Professionalism. If a student is unable to complete a flagged step without cueing, they will need to return at another time to redo the check-off. All other steps can be cued.

Chapter 15

Therapeutic Exercise

Larson T. *Entry-Level Skill Checklists for*
Physical Therapist Assistant Students (pp 169-175).
© 2023 Taylor & Francis Group.

Student Name: _____

Skill		Therapeutic Exercise: Range of Motion			
Source		Klaczak Kopack J, Cascardi KA. *Principles of Therapeutic Exercise for the Physical Therapist Assistant.* SLACK Incorporated; 2023.	**Check When Completed**		
			Self	Peer	Instructor
Student Introduction and Consent	1 ⚑	The student introduces themself to the patient. Must include that they are a **student** PTA and list the school's name.	☐	☐	☐
	2 ⚑	The student verifies the patient's identity. Must use at least 2 patient identifiers (name, date of birth).	☐	☐	☐
	3 ⚑	The student gains consent: • Speaks with the patient about their status (acquires relevant information) • Educates the patient on intended data collection/intervention and goals for the session • Gains permission to perform said data collection/intervention	☐	☐	☐
Student, Patient, and Supply Preparation	4 ⚑	The student gathers supplies and prepares treatment area (cleans equipment, checks for safety hazards, ensures all equipment is functional and appropriate).	☐	☐	☐
	5	The student washes their hands:			
		Student removes all jewelry from their wrists and hands. Student turns the water to the preferred temperature and wets their hands. Student applies the soap to their hands and washes them with their hands pointed down. Student scrubs for 40–60 seconds and includes palm, between fingers, fingernails, and dorsum of hands. Student rinses hands with hands pointed down. Student dries their hands with a paper towel, uses a paper towel to turn off the water, and then disposes of the paper towel in the trash.	☐	☐	☐
	6	The student places the patient in the correct position for support, comfort, and access to body area necessary for data collection/intervention.	☐	☐	☐
Skill Performance	7	The student correctly performs **Passive Range of Motion (PROM)**:			
		Patient is put in a comfortable position that allows full, unrestricted motion at the targeted joint.	☐	☐	☐
		Student uses a firm grasp while fully supporting/cradling the relaxed affected limb.	☐	☐	☐
		Student moves the limb in a slow, rhythmic manner through the available *pain-free* range of motion.	☐	☐	☐
		Student monitors patient carefully throughout the intervention, modifying the technique as needed.	☐	☐	☐
		The limb should not be moved beyond the point of pain or beyond the current available range of motion.	☐	☐	☐
		Student verbalizes the goals of passive range of motion to instructor: *(Reduce the adverse effects of immobilization, reduce pain, maintain tissue mobility, improve circulation, increase synovial fluid movement).*	☐	☐	☐
	8	The student correctly performs **Active Assisted Range of Motion (AAROM)**:			
		Patient is put in a comfortable position that allows full, unrestricted motion at the targeted joint.	☐	☐	☐
		Student carefully monitors and cues patient to ensure that they safely complete as much of the pain-free range as possible by actively contracting the target muscles. Student provides graded assistance through the range when needed.	☐	☐	☐
		Student monitors patient carefully throughout the intervention, modifying the technique as needed.	☐	☐	☐
		Student verbalizes the goals of active assisted range of motion to instructor: *(Actively contract the target muscles through as much of the range of motion as possible without pain).*	☐	☐	☐

⚑ = Critical Safety Element/Professionalism. If a student is unable to complete a flagged step without cueing, they will need to return at another time to redo the check-off. All other steps can be cued.

	9	The student correctly performs **Active Range of Motion (AROM)**:			
		Patient is put in a comfortable position that allows full, unrestricted motion at the targeted joint.	☐	☐	☐
		Student carefully monitors and cues patient to ensure that they safely complete as much of the pain-free range as possible by actively contracting the target muscles.	☐	☐	☐
		Student monitors patient carefully throughout the intervention, modifying the technique as needed.	☐	☐	☐
		Student verbalizes the goals of active range of motion to instructor: *(Develop stronger muscle contractions, increase circulation through active muscle pumping, improve smooth coordinated movements and functional skills).* **Active range of motion does not increase or maintain strength if a muscle is stronger than 3/5.**	☐	☐	☐
Post-Skill	10	The student washes their hands post–skill performance:			
		Student removes all jewelry from their wrists and hands. Student turns the water to the preferred temperature and wets their hands. Student applies the soap to their hands and washes them with their hands pointed down. Student scrubs for 40–60 seconds and includes palm, between fingers, fingernails, and dorsum of hands. Student rinses hands with hands pointed down. Student dries their hands with a paper towel, uses a paper towel to turn off the water, and then disposes of the paper towel in the trash.	☐	☐	☐
	11	The student verbalizes that they will document their session in the note.	☐	☐	☐
Other	12 ⚑	The student has optimal body mechanics during performance of the skill.	☐	☐	☐
	13 ⚑	The student uses appropriate therapeutic touch.	☐	☐	☐
	14	The student is able to complete the check-off in the time allotted.	☐	☐	☐
Communication	15	The student uses language the patient can understand.	☐	☐	☐
	16	The student listens actively to the patient during the session.	☐	☐	☐
	17	The student ensures the patient understands instructions by having the patient teach back or demonstrate.	☐	☐	☐
	18 ⚑	The student demonstrates confidence and provides the patient with clear instruction and cueing.	☐	☐	☐

Peer Name (Printed)		Peer Signature		Date of Peer Review	
Instructor Name (Printed and Signature)	By signing this skills checklist, I am declaring this student competent in the skill described above.			Date of Instructor Review	
NOTES					

⚑ = Critical Safety Element/Professionalism. If a student is unable to complete a flagged step without cueing, they will need to return at another time to redo the check-off. All other steps can be cued.

Student Name: _____

Skill		Therapeutic Exercise: Stretching			
Source		Klaczak Kopack J, Cascardi KA. *Principles of Therapeutic Exercise for the Physical Therapist Assistant.* SLACK Incorporated; 2023.	**Check When Completed**		
			Self	Peer	Instructor
Student Introduction and Consent	1 ⚑	The student introduces themself to the patient. Must include that they are a **student** PTA and list the school's name.	☐	☐	☐
	2 ⚑	The student verifies the patient's identity. Must use at least 2 patient identifiers (name, date of birth).	☐	☐	☐
	3 ⚑	The student gains consent: • Speaks with the patient about their status (acquires relevant information) • Educates the patient on intended data collection/intervention and goals for the session • Gains permission to perform said data collection/intervention	☐	☐	☐
Student, Patient, and Supply Preparation	4 ⚑	The student gathers supplies and prepares treatment area (cleans equipment, checks for safety hazards, ensures all equipment is functional and appropriate).	☐	☐	☐
	5	The student washes their hands:			
		Student removes all jewelry from their wrists and hands. Student turns the water to the preferred temperature and wets their hands. Student applies the soap to their hands and washes them with their hands pointed down. Student scrubs for 40–60 seconds and includes palm, between fingers, fingernails, and dorsum of hands. Student rinses hands with hands pointed down. Student dries their hands with a paper towel, uses a paper towel to turn off the water, and then disposes of the paper towel in the trash.	☐	☐	☐
	6	The student places the patient in the correct position for support, comfort, and access to body area necessary for data collection/intervention.	☐	☐	☐
Skill Performance	7	The student correctly performs **Passive Stretching**:			
		Student determines the most appropriate patient position. The selected body part should be aligned so the structures can be stretched safely and efficiently.	☐	☐	☐
		Student determines which joint/muscle needs to be fixed/stabilized prior to the stretching activity.	☐	☐	☐
		Communicate what patient should feel during the stretch: *(Discomfort and tightness, but not pain).*	☐	☐	☐
		Determine how long the stretch should be maintained: *(Research varies, 30–60 seconds).*	☐	☐	☐
		Student performs the stretch and monitors patient carefully throughout the intervention, modifying the technique as needed.	☐	☐	☐
		Student performs active range of motion/active assisted range of motion into the newly gained range of motion and encourages patient to use the newly available range of motion as much as possible to maintain it.	☐	☐	☐
Post-Skill	8	The student washes their hands post–skill performance:			
		Student removes all jewelry from their wrists and hands. Student turns the water to the preferred temperature and wets their hands. Student applies the soap to their hands and washes them with their hands pointed down. Student scrubs for 40–60 seconds and includes palm, between fingers, fingernails, and dorsum of hands. Student rinses hands with hands pointed down. Student dries their hands with a paper towel, uses a paper towel to turn off the water, and then disposes of the paper towel in the trash.	☐	☐	☐
	9	The student verbalizes that they will document their session in the note.	☐	☐	☐

⚑ = Critical Safety Element/Professionalism. If a student is unable to complete a flagged step without cueing, they will need to return at another time to redo the check-off. All other steps can be cued.

	10 ⚐	The student has optimal body mechanics during performance of the skill.	☐	☐	☐
Other	11 ⚐	The student uses appropriate therapeutic touch.	☐	☐	☐
	12	The student is able to complete the check-off in the time allotted.	☐	☐	☐
Communication	13	The student uses language the patient can understand.	☐	☐	☐
	14	The student listens actively to the patient during the session.	☐	☐	☐
	15	The student ensures the patient understands instructions by having the patient teach back or demonstrate.	☐	☐	☐
	16 ⚐	The student demonstrates confidence and provides the patient with clear instruction and cueing.	☐	☐	☐

Peer Name (Printed)		**Peer Signature**		**Date of Peer Review**	
Instructor Name (Printed and Signature)	By signing this skills checklist, I am declaring this student competent in the skill described above.			**Date of Instructor Review**	
NOTES					

⚐ = Critical Safety Element/Professionalism. If a student is unable to complete a flagged step without cueing, they will need to return at another time to redo the check-off. All other steps can be cued.

Student Name: _____

Skill		Therapeutic Exercise: Strengthening			
Source		Klaczak Kopack J, Cascardi KA. *Principles of Therapeutic Exercise for the Physical Therapist Assistant.* SLACK Incorporated; 2023.	**Check When Completed**		
			Self	Peer	Instructor
Student Introduction and Consent	1 ⚑	The student introduces themself to the patient. Must include that they are a **student** PTA and list the school's name.	☐	☐	☐
	2 ⚑	The student verifies the patient's identity. Must use at least 2 patient identifiers (name, date of birth).	☐	☐	☐
	3 ⚑	The student gains consent: • Speaks with the patient about their status (acquires relevant information) • Educates the patient on intended data collection/intervention and goals for the session • Gains permission to perform said data collection/intervention	☐	☐	☐
Student, Patient, and Supply Preparation	4 ⚑	The student gathers supplies and prepares treatment area (cleans equipment, checks for safety hazards, ensures all equipment is functional and appropriate).	☐	☐	☐
	5	The student washes their hands:			
		Student removes all jewelry from their wrists and hands. Student turns the water to the preferred temperature and wets their hands. Student applies the soap to their hands and washes them with their hands pointed down. Student scrubs for 40–60 seconds and includes palm, between fingers, fingernails, and dorsum of hands. Student rinses hands with hands pointed down. Student dries their hands with a paper towel, uses a paper towel to turn off the water, and then disposes of the paper towel in the trash.	☐	☐	☐
	6	The student places the patient in the correct position for support, comfort, and access to body area necessary for data collection/intervention.	☐	☐	☐
Skill Performance	7	The student correctly performs **Isometric Contraction**:			
		Student correctly verbalizes the goal of isometric contractions: *(Prevent atrophy, develop joint stability, create static strength at selected points in range of motion, increase circulation, and facilitate muscle contraction).*	☐	☐	☐
		Student determines the most appropriate patient position for the selected muscle group.	☐	☐	☐
		Student clearly instructs patient on how to perform the exercise, including form and contraction time: *(6–10 second hold, 10-second rest between contractions).*	☐	☐	☐
		Patient performs the exercise, and student monitors patient carefully throughout the intervention, modifying the technique as needed.	☐	☐	☐
	8	The student correctly performs **Isotonic Contraction**:			
		Student correctly verbalizes the goal of isotonic contractions: *(Improve motor performance, increase strength, increase endurance).*	☐	☐	☐
		Student determines the most appropriate patient position for the selected muscle group.	☐	☐	☐
		Student clearly instructs patient on how to perform the exercise: *(Concentric contraction = the muscle origin and insertion move closer together as the muscle shortens Eccentric contraction = the muscle origin and insertion move further apart as the muscle lengthens in a controlled manner).*	☐	☐	☐
		Patient performs the exercise, and student monitors patient carefully throughout the intervention, modifying the technique as needed.	☐	☐	☐

⚑ = Critical Safety Element/Professionalism. If a student is unable to complete a flagged step without cueing, they will need to return at another time to redo the check-off. All other steps can be cued.

	9	The student correctly performs **Manual Resistance**:			
		Student correctly verbalizes the goal of manual resistance: *(Forces can be applied at different intensities at various points in the range. The amount of resistance is based on patient's ability to resist the applied forces).*	☐	☐	☐
		Student determines the most appropriate patient position for the selected muscle group.	☐	☐	☐
		Student applies appropriate force in correct direction.	☐	☐	☐
		Student performs the exercise and monitors patient carefully throughout the intervention, modifying the technique as needed.	☐	☐	☐
Post-Skill	10	The student washes their hands post–skill performance:			
		Student removes all jewelry from their wrists and hands. Student turns the water to the preferred temperature and wets their hands. Student applies the soap to their hands and washes them with their hands pointed down. Student scrubs for 40–60 seconds and includes palm, between fingers, fingernails, and dorsum of hands. Student rinses hands with hands pointed down. Student dries their hands with a paper towel, uses a paper towel to turn off the water, and then disposes of the paper towel in the trash.	☐	☐	☐
	11	The student verbalizes that they will document their session in the note.	☐	☐	☐
Other	12 ⚑	The student has optimal body mechanics during performance of the skill.	☐	☐	☐
	13 ⚑	The student uses appropriate therapeutic touch.	☐	☐	☐
	14	The student is able to complete the check-off in the time allotted.	☐	☐	☐
Communication	15	The student uses language the patient can understand.	☐	☐	☐
	16	The student listens actively to the patient during the session.	☐	☐	☐
	17	The student ensures the patient understands instructions by having the patient teach back or demonstrate.	☐	☐	☐
	18 ⚑	The student demonstrates confidence and provides the patient with clear instruction and cueing.	☐	☐	☐

Peer Name (Printed)		**Peer Signature**		**Date of Peer Review**	
Instructor Name (Printed and Signature)	By signing this skills checklist, I am declaring this student competent in the skill described above.			**Date of Instructor Review**	
NOTES					

⚑ = Critical Safety Element/Professionalism. If a student is unable to complete a flagged step without cueing, they will need to return at another time to redo the check-off. All other steps can be cued.

Chapter 16

Wound Management

Larson T. *Entry-Level Skill Checklists for*
Physical Therapist Assistant Students (pp 177-183).
© 2023 Taylor & Francis Group.

Student Name: _____

Skill		Wound Management: Isolation Techniques—Handwashing			
Source		Memolo J. *Procedures and Patient Care for the Physical Therapist Assistant.* SLACK Incorporated; 2019.	Check When Completed		
			Self	Peer	Instructor
Oral Question	1	The student correctly lists 5 times when handwashing is necessary: *(Before, during, and after preparing food. Before eating food. Before and after patient care. Before and after treating a wound. After using the toilet. After blowing nose, coughing, or sneezing. After touching an animal, animal food, or animal waste. After touching garbage).*	☐	☐	☐
Supply Preparation	2 ⚑	The student gathers supplies and prepares treatment area (soap, paper towels).	☐	☐	☐
Skill Performance	3	The student correctly performs **Handwashing Procedure**:			
		Student removes all jewelry from their wrists and hands.	☐	☐	☐
		Student turns the water to the preferred temperature and wets their hands.	☐	☐	☐
		Student applies the soap to their hands and washes them with their hands pointed down.	☐	☐	☐
		Student scrubs for 40–60 seconds and includes palm, between fingers, fingernails, and dorsum of hands.	☐	☐	☐
		Student rinses hands with hands pointed down.	☐	☐	☐
		Student dries their hands with a paper towel, uses a paper towel to turn off the water, and then disposes of the paper towel in the trash.	☐	☐	☐
Other	4	The student is able to complete the check-off in the time allotted.	☐	☐	☐
Peer Name (Printed)			Peer Signature		Date of Peer Review	
Instructor Name (Printed and Signature)		By signing this skills checklist, I am declaring this student competent in the skill described above.			Date of Instructor Review	
NOTES					

⚑ = Critical Safety Element/Professionalism. If a student is unable to complete a flagged step without cueing, they will need to return at another time to redo the check-off. All other steps can be cued.

Student Name: _____

Skill		Wound Management: Isolation Techniques—Donning and Doffing Personal Protective Equipment			
Sources		Centers for Disease Control and Prevention. Sequence for putting on personal protective equipment (PPE). Accessed September 14, 2022. https://www.cdc.gov/ hai/pdfs/ppe/PPE-Sequence.pdf Memolo J. *Procedures and Patient Care for the Physical Therapist Assistant.* SLACK Incorporated; 2019.	**Check When Completed**		
			Self	Peer	Instructor
Student, Patient, and Supply Preparation	1 ⚑	The student gathers supplies and prepares treatment area (gown, mask, gloves).	☐	☐	☐
	2	The student washes their hands:			
		Student removes all jewelry from their wrists and hands. Student turns the water to the preferred temperature and wets their hands. Student applies the soap to their hands and washes them with their hands pointed down. Student scrubs for 40–60 seconds and includes palm, between fingers, fingernails, and dorsum of hands. Student rinses hands with hands pointed down. Student dries their hands with a paper towel, uses a paper towel to turn off the water, and then disposes of the paper towel in the trash.	☐	☐	☐
Skill Performance	3	The student correctly **Dons PPE**:			
		Student dons the gown by pulling the sleeve to the wrists and tying the gown behind the neck and around the waist.	☐	☐	☐
		Student dons mask by securing ties or elastic bands at middle of head/neck. Student ensures that the flexible band is fitted to nose bridge and the mask fits snug below chin.	☐	☐	☐
		Student dons their gloves ensuring that the gloves cover the wrist of the isolation gown.	☐	☐	☐
	4	The student correctly **Doffs PPE**:			
		Student doffs gloves by using gloved hand to grasp the palm area of the other gloved hand and peeling off first glove. Student holds removed glove in gloved hand and slides ungloved finger under the remaining glove to peel it off over the first glove. Student disposes of gloves in a waste container.	☐	☐	☐
		Student doffs gown by unfastening gown ties ensuring that sleeves don't contact body when reaching for ties. Student pulls gown away from neck and shoulder touching inside of gown only. Student turns gown inside out and rolls it into a bundle to discard in waste container.	☐	☐	☐
		Student removes mask by grasping bottom ties/elastic and then the top ones ensuring that the front of the mask is not touched. Student then discards mask in waste container.	☐	☐	☐
Post-Skill	5	The student washes their hands post–skill performance:			
		Student removes all jewelry from their wrists and hands. Student turns the water to the preferred temperature and wets their hands. Student applies the soap to their hands and washes them with their hands pointed down. Student scrubs for 40–60 seconds and includes palm, between fingers, fingernails, and dorsum of hands. Student rinses hands with hands pointed down. Student dries their hands with a paper towel, uses a paper towel to turn off the water, and then disposes of the paper towel in the trash.	☐	☐	☐

⚑ = Critical Safety Element/Professionalism. If a student is unable to complete a flagged step without cueing, they will need to return at another time to redo the check-off. All other steps can be cued.

Other	6	The student is able to complete the check-off in the time allotted.			☐	☐	☐
Peer Name (Printed)			**Peer Signature**		**Date of Peer Review**		
Instructor Name (Printed and Signature)	By signing this skills checklist, I am declaring this student competent in the skill described above.				**Date of Instructor Review**		
NOTES							

☐ = Critical Safety Element/Professionalism. If a student is unable to complete a flagged step without cueing, they will need to return at another time to redo the check-off. All other steps can be cued.

Student Name: _____

Skill		Wound Management: Sterile Techniques—Donning and Doffing Sterile Gloves				
Source		Memolo J. *Procedures and Patient Care for the Physical Therapist Assistant.* SLACK Incorporated; 2019.	**Check When Completed**			
			Self	Peer	Instructor	
Student, Patient, and Supply Preparation	1 ⚑	The student gathers supplies and prepares treatment area.	☐	☐	☐	
	2	The student washes their hands:				
		Student removes all jewelry from their wrists and hands. Student turns the water to the preferred temperature and wets their hands. Student applies the soap to their hands and washes them with their hands pointed down. Student scrubs for 40–60 seconds and includes palm, between fingers, fingernails, and dorsum of hands. Student rinses hands with hands pointed down. Student dries their hands with a paper towel, uses a paper towel to turn off the water, and then disposes of the paper towel in the trash.	☐	☐	☐	
Skill Performance	3	The student correctly **Dons Sterile Gloves**:				
		Student opens the sterile glove packet and arranges them so cuffs are facing them without touching the outer surface of the gloves.	☐	☐	☐	
		Student applies the first glove by grasping the cuff that is folded inside out, ensuring not to touch the outer surface of the glove.	☐	☐	☐	
		Student applies the second glove using the now-gloved hand, ensuring to only touch the outside of the glove with the gloved hand. Student slides fingers inside the cuff and pulls glove onto hand.	☐	☐	☐	
	4	The student correctly **Doffs Sterile Gloves**:				
		Student uses gloved hand to pull the other glove inside out, ensuring that they are only touching the outside of the glove.	☐	☐	☐	
		Student uses the ungloved hand and reaches inside the glove to pull it off inside out, ensuring that they are only touching the inside of the glove.	☐	☐	☐	
Post-Skill	5	The student washes their hands post–skill performance:				
		Student removes all jewelry from their wrists and hands. Student turns the water to the preferred temperature and wets their hands. Student applies the soap to their hands and washes them with their hands pointed down. Student scrubs for 40–60 seconds and includes palm, between fingers, fingernails, and dorsum of hands. Student rinses hands with hands pointed down. Student dries their hands with a paper towel, uses a paper towel to turn off the water, and then disposes of the paper towel in the trash.	☐	☐	☐	
Other	6	The student is able to complete the check-off in the time allotted.	☐	☐	☐	
Peer Name (Printed)			**Peer Signature**		**Date of Peer Review**	
Instructor Name (Printed and Signature)		By signing this skills checklist, I am declaring this student competent in the skill described above.			**Date of Instructor Review**	
NOTES						

⚑ = Critical Safety Element/Professionalism. If a student is unable to complete a flagged step without cueing, they will need to return at another time to redo the check-off. All other steps can be cued.

Student Name: _____

Skill		Wound Management: Sterile Techniques—Application of a Wound Dressing and Sterile Field			
Source		Memolo J. *Procedures and Patient Care for the Physical Therapist Assistant.* SLACK Incorporated; 2019.	**Check When Completed**		
			Self	Peer	Instructor
Student Introduction and Consent	1 ⚑	The student introduces themself to the patient. Must include that they are a **student** PTA and list the school's name.	☐	☐	☐
	2 ⚑	The student verifies the patient's identity. Must use at least 2 patient identifiers (name, date of birth).	☐	☐	☐
	3 ⚑	The student gains consent: • Speaks with the patient about their status (acquires relevant information) • Educates the patient on intended data collection/intervention and goals for the session • Gains permission to perform said data collection/intervention	☐	☐	☐
Student, Patient, and Supply Preparation	4 ⚑	The student gathers supplies and prepares treatment area (cleans equipment, checks for safety hazards, ensures all equipment is functional and appropriate).	☐	☐	☐
	5	The student washes their hands:			
		Student removes all jewelry from their wrists and hands. Student turns the water to the preferred temperature and wets their hands. Student applies the soap to their hands and washes them with their hands pointed down. Student scrubs for 40–60 seconds and includes palm, between fingers, fingernails, and dorsum of hands. Student rinses hands with hands pointed down. Student dries their hands with a paper towel, uses a paper towel to turn off the water, and then disposes of the paper towel in the trash.	☐	☐	☐
	6	The student places the patient in the correct position for support, comfort, and access to body area necessary for data collection/intervention.	☐	☐	☐
Skill Performance	7	The student correctly **Sets Up a Sterile Field**:			
		Student opens the sterile towel packaging, ensuring to only touch the outer 1 inch of the drape.	☐	☐	☐
		Student places the unopened packages of required supplies near the sterile field, but not on it.	☐	☐	☐
		Student opens sterile utensils over the sterile field and drops them onto the sterile towel.	☐	☐	☐
	8	The student correctly **Applies a Wound Dressing**:			
		Student cleanses the wound as directed by therapist's plan of care.	☐	☐	☐
		Student applies the contact layer (medication, petroleum jelly, etc)	☐	☐	☐
		Student applies the intermediate layer (gauze, sponge, pad, etc)	☐	☐	☐
		Student applies the outer layer (Kerlix, Ace wrap, Tubigrip, etc) ensuring that the tension is not so much to occlude blood flow.	☐	☐	☐
Post-Skill	9	The student washes their hands post–skill performance:			
		Student removes all jewelry from their wrists and hands. Student turns the water to the preferred temperature and wets their hands. Student applies the soap to their hands and washes them with their hands pointed down. Student scrubs for 40–60 seconds and includes palm, between fingers, fingernails, and dorsum of hands. Student rinses hands with hands pointed down. Student dries their hands with a paper towel, uses a paper towel to turn off the water, and then disposes of the paper towel in the trash.	☐	☐	☐
	10	The student verbalizes that they will document their session in the note.	☐	☐	☐

⚑ = Critical Safety Element/Professionalism. If a student is unable to complete a flagged step without cueing, they will need to return at another time to redo the check-off. All other steps can be cued.

Other	11 ⚑	The student has optimal body mechanics during performance of the skill.	☐	☐	☐
	12 ⚑	The student uses appropriate therapeutic touch.	☐	☐	☐
	13	The student is able to complete the check-off in the time allotted.	☐	☐	☐
Communication	14	The student uses language the patient can understand.	☐	☐	☐
	15	The student listens actively to the patient during the session.	☐	☐	☐
	16	The student ensures the patient understands instructions by having the patient teach back or demonstrate.	☐	☐	☐
	17 ⚑	The student demonstrates confidence and provides the patient with clear instruction and cueing.	☐	☐	☐
Peer Name (Printed)			**Peer Signature**		**Date of Peer Review**	
Instructor Name (Printed and Signature)	By signing this skills checklist, I am declaring this student competent in the skill described above.				**Date of Instructor Review**	
NOTES					

⚑ = Critical Safety Element/Professionalism. If a student is unable to complete a flagged step without cueing, they will need to return at another time to redo the check-off. All other steps can be cued.

REFERENCES

Centers for Disease Control and Prevention. Sequence for putting on personal protective equipment (PPE). Accessed September 14, 2022. https://www.cdc.gov/hai/pdfs/ppe/PPE-Sequence.pdf

Klaczak Kopack J, Cascardi KA. *Principles of Therapeutic Exercise for the Physical Therapist Assistant.* SLACK Incorporated; 2023.

Lazaro RT, Umphred DA. *Umphred's Neurorehabilitation for the Physical Therapist Assistant.* 3rd ed. SLACK Incorporated; 2021.

Memolo J. *Procedures and Patient Care for the Physical Therapist Assistant.* SLACK Incorporated; 2019.

Memolo J. *Therapeutic Agents for the Physical Therapist Assistant.* SLACK Incorporated; 2022.

Physical Therapy. Education. Redefined. PhysioU. Accessed September 14, 2022. https://www.physiou.health/

Van Ost L, Morogiello J. *Cram Session in Goniometry and Manual Muscle Testing: A Handbook for Students & Clinicians.* 2nd ed. SLACK Incorporated; 2023.

Printed in the United States
by Baker & Taylor Publisher Services